THE WOMAN PATIENT

Volume 2
Concepts of Femininity
and the Life Cycle

WOMEN IN CONTEXT: Development and Stresses

THE WOMAN PATIENT
> *Volume 1: Sexual and Reproductive Aspects of Women's Health Care*
> Edited by Malkah T. Notman and Carol C. Nadelson

> *Volume 2: Concepts of Femininity and the Life Cycle*
> Edited by Carol C. Nadelson and Malkah T. Notman

> *Volume 3: Aggression, Adaptations, and Psychotherapy*
> Edited by Malkah T. Notman and Carol C. Nadelson

BECOMING FEMALE: PERSPECTIVES ON DEVELOPMENT
> Edited by Claire B. Kopp

WOMEN'S SEXUAL DEVELOPMENT: EXPLORATIONS OF INNER SPACE
> Edited by Martha Kirkpatrick

WOMEN'S SEXUAL EXPERIENCE: EXPLORATIONS OF THE
DARK CONTINENT
> Edited by Martha Kirkpatrick

THE WOMAN PATIENT

Volume 2
Concepts of Femininity and the Life Cycle

EDITED BY

CAROL C. NADELSON, M. D.

AND

MALKAH T. NOTMAN, M. D.

Tufts University School of Medicine
Boston, Massachusetts

PLENUM PRESS · NEW YORK AND LONDON

Library of Congress Cataloging in Publication Data

Main entry under title:

Concepts of femininity and the life cycle.
  (The woman patient; v. 2) (Women in context)
  Bibliography: p.
  Includes index.
  Contents: Feminine development / Malkah Notman—Changing views of the relation-
ship beetween femininity and reproduction / Malkah Notman and Carol Nadelson—
Changing sex stereotypes / Norman E. Zinber—[etc.]
  1. Women—Mental health—Addresses, essays, lectures. 2. Femininity (Psychology)
—Addresses, essays, lectures. 3. Women—Psychology—Addresses, essays, lectures. I.
Nadelson, Carol C. II. Notman, Malkah T. III. Series. IV. Series: Women in context.
[DNLM: 1. Delivery of health care. 2. Genital diseases, Female. 3. Women. WP 100.3
W872 1978]
RC451.4.W6C66   616.89′0088042   82-5326
ISBN-13: 978-1-4615-9244-0   e-ISBN-13: 978-1-4615-9242-6   AACR2
DOI: 10.1007/978-1-4615-9242-6

©1982 Plenum Press, New York
Softcover reprint of the hardcover 1st edition 1982
A Division of Plenum Publishing Corporation
233 Spring Street, New York, N.Y. 10013

Contributors

T. Berry Brazelton, M.D. ● Associate Chief of Pediatrics, Harvard Medical School; Chief of Child Development Unit, Children's Hospital Medical Center, Boston, Massachusetts

Golda M. Edinburg, ACSW ● Director, Social Work Department, McLean Hospital, Belmont, Massachusetts

Constance H. Keefer, M.D. ● Pediatrician, Harvard Community Health Plan; Clinical Instructor, Pediatrics, Harvard Medical School, Boston, Massachusetts

Mary Alice Mathews, M.D. ● Clinical Instructor in Psychiatry, Harvard Medical School; Assistant in Psychiatry, Beth Israel Hospital, Boston, Massachusetts

Carol Nadelson, M.D. ● Professor and Vice-chairman, Department of Psychiatry; Director of Training and Education, Tufts University School of Medicine-New England Medical Center Hospital, Boston, Massachusetts

Malkah Notman, M.D. ● Director, Women's Resource Center, Clinical Professor of Psychiatry, Tufts University School of Medicine-New England Medical Center Hospital, Boston, Massachusetts

Derek C. Polonsky, M.D. ● Director, Family Institute, New England Medical Center; Assistant Clinical Professor, Tufts University School of Medicine, Boston, Massachusetts

Joan J. Zilbach, M.D. ● Director, Family Therapy and Research, Judge Baker Guidance Center; Senior Training Consultant and Supervisor, Child and Family Program, Boston Veterans Administration Hospital, Boston, Massachusetts

Veva H. Zimmerman, M.D. ● Associate Dean and Associate Professor of Clinical Psychiatry, New York University School of Medicine, New York

Norman E. Zinberg, M.D. • Clinical Professor of Psychiatry, Harvard Medical School, The Cambridge Hospital, Cambridge, Massachusetts

Preface

In Volumes 2 and 3, we have chosen a focus that places in context aspects of mental health and the complex psychosocial factors that affect our perceptions of how health and illness are defined and experienced.

We are aware that some may take exceptions to the topics chosen or to the way in which some authors have developed their ideas and presented their information. While we cannot expect to agree with each other all of the time, we can provide a framework and a perspective from which ideas can take form and evolve.

The first section of Volume 2 provides an overview of some of the theoretical issues involved in understanding the psychology of women. These issues include changes in psychoanalytic views, particularly in relation to femininity and feminine development. The particular developmental experiences of black women are also clearly delineated. The second section deals with specific points in the life cycle that raise unique issues for women, especially as they pertain to the many roles of women in contemporary society and the impact that these roles have on their careers and on their families. The impact of having a working mother on the early interaction with children, the concerns of midlife, especially marital interactions, and the ambiguities of aging are discussed.

We intend to provide information and to raise questions that we hope will be part of an ongoing dialogue, as well as a stimulus to more intensive study and understanding.

We would like to thank our families, for their support, contributions, and understanding, and our editor, Hilary Evans, for her patience and endurance. We are also grateful for the contributing authors' hard work and tolerance during the process of writing and rewriting.

CAROL C. NADELSON
MALKAH T. NOTMAN

Boston, Massachusetts
November, 1981

vii

Contents

PART I

Theory

Chapter 1

Feminine Development: Changes in Psychoanalytic Theory

MALKAH NOTMAN

Psychoanalysis does not represent a unified, static body of theory or practice; rather, it has changed constantly. Since the original discoveries of Freud, developments and modifications have been continual in all areas of psychoanalysis: theory, research, and therapy. Psychoanalytic theory about women has also undergone many changes. Although many of Freud's patients were women, and he paid attention to disorders and complaints that other physicians dismissed, his theories have been seen as critical and demeaning of women. Since many of the original formulations were developed in the culture of Freud's time, they reflected the phallocentric aspects of that culture. With the exceptions of criticism and modifications by Karen Horney,[1] Ernest Jones,[2] and later some few others, such as Clara Thompson[3] and Gregory Zilboorg,[4] the ideas were rarely questioned from positions outside that culture until recently, when psychoanalytic views about women have received particular attention and have been subject to considerable changes, partly in response to impact of the women's movement.

It is interesting to note the extent to which the male's development and psychic structure were considered central to the theoretical formulations, which described human development from the point of view of the male. The female's developmental path was then examined as a "variant" of the male's. This has been true in all areas of psychology.[5,6,7,8] Freud did explicitly state that he thought he did not understand women well, and he stressed the need for knowledge about

MALKAH NOTMAN, M.D. • Department of Psychiatry, Tufts University-New England Medical Center Hospital, Boston, Massachusetts.

women's biology and psychology.[9] Freud presented some excellent clinical descriptions that were based on his and others' observations. However, he drew a particular set of conclusions from those observations, as if these conclusions were also universally valid. It is possible to draw alternative conclusions from these same observations that are not as influenced by the same cultural stereotypes, but that take into account the impact of socialization on what were thought to be innate processes and that also include a more contemporary understanding of biology and development.

Psychoanalysis is still identified by some as a field that depreciates women. However, important advances in understanding women have also been made, and there have been a number of recent contributors who have reexamined old ideas and made major revisions. Early formulations were frequently based on inferences and reconstructions of child development from clinical experience with adults. Many of these have since been replaced by concepts based on observations of actual child development, in "normal" as well as patient populations. In recent years, careful observations of very young infants have also contributed to major revisions in human-development and psychoanalytic theory. Modern technical advances have made more sophisticated tools available for observation and experimentation in the biological sciences and related fields. The disciplines of biology, anthropology, and sociology were not as well developed in the period of Freud's first writing and have contributed further new data.

In this chapter, I shall address several major classical concepts about femininity and feminine development and indicate the changes that have occurred in contemporary psychoanalysis. First, I shall present a discussion of "femininity," with a review of the ideas of Freud and other classical analysts about the concepts of passivity, masochism, narcissism, penis envy, and bisexuality, which have become such pivotal terms in the discussion of femininity; then, I shall relate more current evidence to this material and finally conclude with some contemporary ideas about feminine development.

CONCEPTS OF FEMININITY

Femininity is very difficult to define because the word is used in a number of ways. It can be used descriptively, normatively, diagnostically, clinically, and colloquially. The confusion of the descriptive and normative uses has long been a problem.[10] When one attempts to focus on what might be the "essential" components, even from a descriptive point of view, one encounters the problem of drawing boundaries between the effects of socialization and inherent biological determinants. It is clear from many studies of the very early postnatal interactions of caretakers and infants that parental expectations related to the gender of the infant affect the behavior of the caretakers toward the infant.[11,12] Socialization begins at this very early period. Infant development is now understood to be a reciprocal process in which the infant stimulates responses in the caretaker as well as being cared for.

The descriptive norms of femininity are often difficult to separate from the proscriptive ones. An illustration is the finding that many women are indeed more passive and less manifestly aggressive than most men. This is clinically true; at the same time, this pattern probably also represents an expression of lifelong restrictions against expressing aggression and activity directly and indirectly, as well as against being self-assertive in achieving one's own goals, in circumstances where self-assertion is considered appropriate for males.[13]

It may be more appropriate to regard *femininity* as a variable concept with mutually interacting influences and determinants from genetic, anatomical, and instinctual sources, as well as from interpersonal and social forces. Being born a girl, therefore, means coming into the world as an individual with a specific genetic endowment and specific anatomical structures, with the potential for their further development in a recognized feminine direction, under the influence of specific hormones. These hormones are present prenatally and postnatally and continually influence the developmental process. At the same time, being born a girl activates specific expectations in parents and others and stimulates responses that are different in many ways from those that are aroused toward a boy baby.[11,12,14] These responses are culturally determined as well as having their origins in each individual's personal and family history. In turn, all these influences affect the shaping of the baby into someone who eventually looks like and behaves as a "feminine" person.

Freud's and Others' Early Concepts of Femininity

Freud's original description of femininity, which was further elaborated by Helene Deutsch, involved a triad of characteristics: passivity, masochism, and narcissism.[15] Freud's original formulation also characterized femininity as giving preference to "passive aims,"[16] which he distinguished from passivity itself, saying that to achieve a passive aim may demand a great deal of activity, and he thus acknowledged the activity involved in maternal behavior. Although he warned against equating masculinity with activity and femininity with passivity, he himself did not heed the warning and often used *passive* for "feminine" and *active* for "masculine."

To understand the differences between men and women, Freud turned to their early development. He believed that girls and boys develop similarly for the first three years, until they became fully aware of the anatomical differences between them. He thought that children assumed that everyone started life with the same form of genital (i.e., a penis), and that the discovery of the female body with the "missing" genital constituted a "castration shock" for both boys and girls. The girl thought she had had a penis originally and had lost it, for which she blamed her mother and felt angry, envious, and defective. This Freud saw as a turning point in the little girl's growth. He viewed her early development as essentially "masculine" and her pleasurable sexual sensations as deriving from her clitoris as parallel to the boy's phallic experiences. The girl's early masturbation was also viewed as "masculine" because it was thought to be primarily clitoral. Her early relationship with her mother was profoundly affected by this discovery of her "inferiority" and her disappointment.

Freud believed that these feelings of inferiority led to the little girl's temporary renunciation of sexuality. It is important to remember that Freud was the first to recognize the importance of infantile sexuality and of masturbation as part of the development of normal sexual feelings and their expression. He discussed masturbation and its significance in relation to three phases: an infantile phase, a childhood phase, and then a new phase in adolescence. He believed that early masturbation in girls was clitoral and not vaginal. This concept also entered into the understanding of the body image of the girl, that is, how the girl viewed herself and her body, and particularly her genitals. Since he thought of the clitoris as an inferior, small penis, he assumed that the little girl experienced it in the same way and that she inevitably felt disappointed. As a consequence of this disappointment, she renounced some of her sexuality, and at least some of her masturbation as well.[9,17,18]

PASSIVITY. Another important consequence of this experience was that the little girl turned away from her mother, whom she also devalued, as she realized that her mother did not have a penis either, and she turned toward her father and began her Oedipus complex (or Electra complex, as others have referred to this phase in women). In this process, her earlier activity was given up and passivity gained the upper hand, leading her eventually to give up the wish for a penis and to substitute the wish for a baby in the course of her development toward femininity.

These ideas about feminine development were shared by other

analysts, although they were challenged to some extent by Karen Horney and Ernest Jones.[1,2] Jones, Klein, and some others stressed the relationship between the girl and her mother, which, they believed, played a preponderant role in the child's life in the first year.[19] They also thought that the little girl started out "more feminine than masculine," rather than following Freud's formulation.

Freud and other early analysts believed that the little girl was really not aware of her inner genital organs nor of her vagina and did not integrate these into her self-image, and that therefore she could not create a positive feeling about her anatomy.[17] In the change that was to occur later for the girl when sexual feelings shifted from the clitoris to the vagina, Freud saw a renunciation of the "early masculine phase" of femininity, or the "childish masculinity," and this shift from clitoris to vagina was part of feminine development. Little girls were therefore thought of as if they were "castrated" boys, and femininity was consolidated only after a period of disappointment with themselves. The wish for a baby, an important component of feminine identity, was therefore thought to be a replacement for what the girl did not have. The enormous personal development necessary for successful parenthood and its positive experience were not considered at this point.

It was thought, therefore, that the castration complex and penis envy motivated the girl's turning away from her mother and toward her father. In boys, the Oedipal development was different. The growing sexualized attachment to the mother and the consequent rivalry with the father intensified the little boy's anxiety and fear of punishment. He developed "castration anxiety" as a result of learning about sex differences, and he interpreted the girl's lack of a penis as the result of castration, which he then feared for himself. Castration anxiety constituted a powerful motivation for renouncing his Oedipal wishes for his mother and thus for his movement out of the Oedipal phase.

In attempting to understand femininity as well as the role of reproduction and the genitals, divergent psychoanalytic theories about feminine development centered for a time on this question of whether early vaginal sensations existed, and whether the little girl was aware of the vagina and the uterus as organs that could contain a baby.[20] Those who believed that she *did* have this awareness also assumed an early development of what was considered femininity. Although there was some disagreement about the details of this process, pregnancy and mothering, the awareness of the vagina, and the expectation of future babies were seen as central to feminine identity.

Other psychoanalysts, such as Benedek[21] and Bonaparte,[22] sought some further explanation for women's drive organization and maternal behavior and turned to biological and instinctual determinants. Benedek thought that the major basis for the biological roots of the feelings associated with pregnancy and motherhood was to be found in the fluctuation of the female endocrine cycle. She studied this cycle and concluded that the "deep rooted passivity" and "tendency toward introversion" described by Helene Deutsch[15] as characteristic of the female psyche appeared mostly in connection with the postovulative phase of the menstrual cycle. She also looked for some connections between feminine characteristics and cyclical changes and studied hormonal variations and psychological material, attempting to establish relationships using the relatively crude hormonal assays of the 1940s. She thought she did find connections between cyclic menstrual phases and variations in psychic states, and she concluded that "the emotional manifestations of the 'specific receptive tendency' and the 'self-centered retentive tendency' are the psychodynamic correlates of a biologic need for motherhood"; and therefore, Benedek saw motherhood not as secondary or as a substitute for the missing penis, but as "the manifestation of an instinct for survival in the child that is the primary organizer of the woman's sexual drive and her personality."[23] In this, she anticipated current writers who stress the nonsubstitutive nature of the wish for a child and who describe the reciprocal nature of the development of motherly feelings as a response to the infant's needs.[24,25,26] Although developmental identification with one's mother was seen by Benedek and others as an important determinant of a woman's emotional attitude toward motherhood and of her mothering behavior, the central role of the pre-Oedipal identification with the mother was not emphasized as much by earlier writers as was the biological, if not the instinctual, origin of mothering behavior and of the female drive organization. Adult women's psychological attitudes were thought to be dependent on a hormonal or some other biological origin and the idea of the wish for a baby as a replacement for the organ she did not have was prevalent in the literature.

MASOCHISM. A second component of the feminine triad was masochism, which Freud saw as being due to "the suppression of women's aggressiveness which is prescribed for them constitutionally and imposed on them socially which favors the development of powerful masochistic impulses." He went on to say that masochism was "truly feminine."[9]

The early literature contained some discussion of whether masochism was biologically determined or inherent in the feminine personality and whether feminine masochism represented an adaptation to the inevitable pain of childbearing or other essentially feminine experiences.[27] Helene Deutsch considered "feminine masochism" parallel to "activity directed inward."[15] It was thought that a woman's masochism was parallel to the man's intensified aggression, which accompanied his activity directed "outward" at the end of adolescence. Deutsch thus distinguished feminine masochism from the neurotic masochism that manifested itself in perversions and neurotic suffering and pain. She spoke instead of a passive-masochistic character type characterizing the normal feminine psychological structure. Recent theoretical formulations have questioned this view and will be discussed later in this chapter.

NARCISSISM. The third element in the classical feminine triad was narcissism. The concept of narcissism has acquired different contemporary meanings, relating to descriptions and diagnoses of personality types. These are not discussed here. In describing feminine narcissism, Freud said "thus we attribute a larger amount of narcissism to femininity, which also affects women's choice of object, so that to be loved is a stronger need for them than to love,"[9,15] and "the effect of penis envy has a share in the physical vanity of women, since they are bound to value their charms more highly as a late compensation for their original sexual inferiority."[9] Freud was both describing clinical phenomena and ascribing dynamic reasons for them in these statements. It was a narcissistic disappointment that, according to Freud, led the little girl to withdraw from her mother when she discovered her lack of a penis, and then to turn to her father. Freud described "feminine love [as] passive and narcissistic," so that the woman "lets herself be loved."

It is clear from what has been said that although Freud respected individual women, valued them as colleagues, and was one of the first physicians to take many baffling problems of women seriously, he really did feel that many "feminine" characteristics were due to an actual genital inferiority, which women also believed themselves, and that the consequence of this inferiority was the need to overcome or hide these facts. He thought a woman was fully satisfied only when she had a son, compensating for her penis envy and feelings of inferiority. The greater cultural value and status of a male child over a female child as a reason for the possible preference of a male did not seem to be considered in his arguments.

CONTEMPORARY PSYCHOANALYTIC THINKING

There have been successive changes in the formulations about women and their development and psychology.[28] Questions and modifications came from within the psychoanalytic movement in its early days, and later from data from other fields and from the evolution of thinking as social changes had an impact on sex roles, family patterns, and other social realities.

Recent writers have brought forward evidence to clarify feminine development and to challenge some of the early psychoanalytic views. The images of women as anatomically defective because of the absence of the penis and the substitutive nature of childbearing, for example, have been questioned extensively.[28,29,30] For example, Chasseguet-Smirgel says, "Images of women as deficient or castrated are a denial for both sexes of the images of the primitive mother, the good omnipotent mother, symbolized by the generous breast, fruitful womb, wholeness, abundance."[7]

Many recent authors have addressed themselves to the question of feminine identity, its sources in childhood, and its manifestations during a girl's growing up and have attempted to create a concept of femininity and an understanding of feminine development based on knowledge of the female course of development rather than on a reliance on the model of the male as the starting point. However, the components of femininity are not uniformly agreed on. Even the role of reproduction has not been consistently conceptualized in relation to "femininity."

In attempting to arrive at a contemporary definition of femininity, one must include a number of components. One set consists of those behaviors, attitudes, and styles presented as feminine in a given culture. Those are, in turn, related to physical functions that are exclusively female, such as reproduction, and any other behaviors and feelings dynamically related to these reproductive roles. One may ask whether it is necessary to have a sharp dichotomy between what is considered "masculine" or "feminine." Although many distinctions between masculine and feminine behavior are blurring, and there may be fewer inherent differences between the capacities of men and women than used to be thought, there do appear to be some differences.

Recent research in neurobiology has begun to shed some light on the interaction of genetic endowment; maturational state, rate, and patterns; and apparent masculine–feminine differences. In the past, differences between men and women have been used to justify inequities. This has led to some attempts to minimize differences, thereby to create more social justice. However, some tendency to polarize masculine and feminine does seem to exist in all cultures. Perhaps this tendency is more limited in some countries than it was in the past, but it is hard to assess these changes at present. To some extent, role distinctions and polarization derive from the male–female differences related to childbearing, which demands that the woman tolerate a pregnancy and the resulting ambiguous boundary between herself and another human being. Women have also been most responsible for the care of young children and its many moments of closeness, which may be derived from the intimacy of pregnancy. The early differences between boys' and girls' relationships to their male and female parents may also be an important basis of a developmentally different outcome. For example, in separating himself from an early attachment and initial identification with a female parent, the little boy must differentiate himself from the feminine personality,[28] and in resisting that regressive attachment, he may assert a sharper "masculinity."

It is therefore difficult to describe femininity without including some reference to the reproductive functions of the woman and the identification with and anticipation of these by the little girl. It is also difficult to discuss femininity apart from masculinity, a concept that has also been changing in recent years. Questions have been raised about whether a woman's self-esteem must be as closely bound up with her attractiveness and relationships to men as it has been, or whether having children will actually be achieved by all women in a period of declining birth rates. Recent concepts seek to define femininity in terms that do not use as a basis the idea that a baby is a substitute for a defect that the girl feels she has, such as the "missing penis"; rather, these concepts seek to delineate a separate line of feminine development. However, reproductive capacity and choice do seem to be important components of femininity in a developing girl, whether or not that choice is actually exercised by an adult woman.

There is also considerable evidence that women do value their relationships to others in a different way than men. They make the kinds of choices that preserve relationships, and they have a sense of responsibility and attachment that is different than that of most men.[5,31] These are important components of the feminine personality. As will be seen later, women handle aggression, anger, and assertion differently than men, and whether these are socialized responses or represent some interweaving of environmental with innate tendencies, there are manifest differences in style.

DATA FROM THE BIOLOGICAL SCIENCES

It is obvious that men and women are anatomically and biologically different. The extent to which the behavioral and the personality differences that accompany sex roles are biologically determined is far from resolved. The role of hormones and the developmental consequences of anatomical differences need to be studied further. Manifest gender differences are generally the result of interactions between the biological determinants and social factors.

However, there are clear maturational and neurological differences from birth; for example, girls are born more mature neurologically. Maturation in a number of areas is also reported to be earlier in girls, and the consequent behavioral and skill differences, in turn, elicit different responses from their caretakers.[32] The implications of these differences for later development are not entirely possible to establish at this date.

Freud believed that "bisexuality" was a constitutional biological potential on which later psychological development rests, and that it was characteristic of all individuals to have both "masculine" and "feminine" traits, although he did not clearly define these.[17,33] Data from studies of embryological development have seemed to confirm this idea, since the reproductive organs of each sex develop from undifferentiated precursors and, in the presence of hormones of the appropriate sex, can appear to develop into either male or female organs. Actually, it is the genetic composition that determines the real sex of the individual: the presence of two X chromosomes is the genetic pattern of females, and the presence of an X and a Y chromosome is the pattern of males. However, the potential exists for modifying the cells, tissues, and organs of each sex in the direction of the opposite sex by introducing appropriate hormones, so that although an individual is genetically female, for instance, circulating male hormones have caused changes in the external genitalia to make her appear male.[34]

The mechanisms of the differentiation into male and female are interesting. The genetic composition of XX or XY determines the initial differentiation of ovary or testis from the primitive, undifferentiated reproductive tissue. The circulating hormones produced by these organs in the fetus then, in turn, determine further differentiation into recognizable sex organs. If the embryo is to be male, the testis differentiates earlier than the ovary and secretes both androgen and a hormone that produces regression of the Müllerian duct system (the precursor of the female organs). In the absence of androgens, the fetus appears female, even though genetically it may be male. Rather than regarding this phenomenon as "bisexuality," more recent investigators have changed the concept to one of "sexual bipotentiality."[33,34] The resting or undifferentiated primary state of mammalian organisms is female. If a male is to be produced from this primary state, androgens must be present at a particular time in fetal development. It is thus possible to have an individual who is genetically male but appears female, in that the external genitalia are undeveloped, and the penis looks like a clitoris. In another abnormal condition, a genetic female has circulating male hormones and may have primitive ovaries and uterus, but because of the growth of the external genitals, she appears male. There are some central-nervous-system effects of these fetal hormones as well, such as changes that are precursors of cycling in the female, leading in later life to menstrual cycles under the subsequent influence of the hypothalamic-pituitary-ovarian interrelationships.

The full implications of these data for psychological development are not immediately apparent. However, they do represent a contrast to the point of view in which normal female development is seen as deriving from that of the male. Research in this area is continuing, and there are many new findings.

GENDER IDENTITY AND ITS RELATION TO "FEMININITY"

The establishment of gender identity has been clarified and distinguished from femininity or masculinity. This concept involves the cognitive awareness of the sex one is. In rare instances, this concept varies from one's "true" sex, as the phenotype may be different from the genotype, because an endocrine or anatomical problem distorts the genitals as seen at birth, and the sex that the infant is labelled (called the *sex of assignment*), which is the sex in which a child is reared, exerts a predominant influence on the individual's self-concept. Gender identity development is accompanied by awareness of sex roles, that is, the behaviors, attitudes, expectations, and appearance that accompany each sex. It is firmly established by about 18 months.[35] Stoller sees this development as untraumatic and unconflicted. He speaks of "primary femininity" as representing the first stage in female development.[34] It consists of the establishment of a sense of being "rightfully a female" and is based on a combination of biological determinants: the sex assignment made at birth, which results in appropriate parental behavior, and also the effects of early postnatal experiences, including bodily sensations, especially from the genitals. He believes that the second stage of feminine development is the result of conflict, particularly Oedipal conflict, the resolution of which produces a more complicated and richer femininity. This idea of a "primary femininity" has gained considerable acceptance.

EARLY DEVELOPMENT AND RELATIONSHIPS

The importance of the early pre-Oedipal attachment to the mother has received increased recognition, supporting some of the early ideas of Jones and Klein, but with some different emphases.[2,19] There is also acknowledgment of the degree and the significance of the little girl's early attachment to her father. Abelin stated that the little girl has a differentiated relationship to the father before her first birthday, between 8 and 18 months.[36] Little girls tend to be generally more discriminating than little boys with regard to unfamiliar persons. Observations of children who are 10–18 months old indicated that the mother is perceived as the expressive affectional parent and the father as the "instrumental" parent.[37] This finding confirms the establishment of the awareness of sex-role differences early, as well as the awareness of the sex-role stereotyping of the predominant styles of women and men.

The importance of infant development is better understood in current theory, and the contribution of pre-Oedipal experience in general is acknowledged more fully. The importance of these pre-Oedipal relationships, before the conflicts of the phallic phase emerge, have been recently reviewed by Galenson.[38] The girl's identification with her mother forms an important early component of her feminine identity, and her sense of gender identity is partly based on this identification. The impact of external reality and of relationships with others on development has been increasingly recognized.

Pre-Oedipal as well as Oedipal experiences and interactions differ for boys and girls. Their relationship to the mother is necessarily different. The mother's relationship with her own mother is re-created by having a daughter. This experience also enables her to identify with her own child and to reexperience the past as well as to make restitution for it, perhaps, by becoming a better mother and daughter.[15,19,39,40] There is likely to be a different, and perhaps more intense, tie between a mother and a daughter than between a mother and a son.[40] This tie had been less emphasized in the past than the importance of the son in supplying the "missing penis." This process of close identification with the daughter may result, however, in increased difficulty for the mother in permitting and supporting differentiation and separation–individuation in her daughter, and there may be a resultant persistence of the strong early attachments to the mother. This phenomenon has been described by many psychoanalytic writers.[2,9,15,41] Chodorow[42] pointed to aspects of the difference in male and female development that may partly account for the affective and relational identifications between women and their mothers as opposed to the kind of identifications that boys have with their fathers, which involve relating more to their status and role. Chodorow feels that the close tie that has been established and the availability of the mother is an important factor. The father, less available in traditionally organized families, is defined more by fantasy and by values and behavior. Because of this difference and the potential regressive appeal of the mother, boys may need more to reject the feminine in order to preserve their masculine identification. In Chodorow's view the identification with the father is strengthened by avoidance of the feminine. Whether the differences between men and women regarding separation and individuation are problems or differences depends on one's point of view. Autonomy may be more difficult, but maintaining important ties and commitments to others also has considerable positive value.[5,31] The role of pregnancy and of the early interactions between mother and infant in the predominance of the mother's early child care is also receiving attention.[43]

THE SIGNIFICANCE OF BODY IMAGE

An additional set of important developmental influences derives from the experience of having a female body, with an opening, rather than the protruding genitals.[34] Girls are brought up with expectations of their inner potential, which are learned later; that is, they know that they are capable of bearing children. They also expect body changes later, including the growth of a new structure, the breasts. This knowledge and this expectation also form part of the feminine self-concept. Although both boys and girls know that their bodies will change as they mature, the capacity to bring forth new life has a greater impact on the female, who will carry it intimately. Certain personality traits that are measured by psychological tests, such as women's tendency to make less sharp differentiations of figure–ground perceptions, and women's greater dependence on and investment in relationships and greater "affiliativeness," may also be subtly influenced by these anatomical differences and their personal implications. For example, the expectation of being connected intimately to another human being who is internal and invisible is congruent with an integration of context into the perception of a figure. To say that there are potential biological influences does not minimize the powerful socializing factors that affect boys and girls from their earliest days.[12,44]

SEX DIFFERENCES IN REARING

An important area of recent research is the documentation of sex differences in the rearing of children, not only when they are toddlers and of school age but from birth on. Even prenatal parental expectations are different for boys and girls. Although Freud was obviously aware that parents treat little girls and boys differently, it has been only in the past 15–20 years that a considerable literature has developed that indicates the extent, depth, subtlety, and significance of these differences. For example, Moss observed infants and mothers over the first three months of life and found profound sex differences in maternal behavior and pronounced shifts from the way the infants were treated at three weeks to the way they were treated at three months.[44] He felt that initially, conditions are set by the infant, with its state—such as fussing, sleeping, and waking—creating an important variable. He found that mothers initially responded more to male infants, who were more irritable. By three months, the mothers were responding less to them and more contingently to females; as a result, he thought, females would be "more amenable to the effects of social reinforcement and manifest a higher degree of attachment behavior." In another study, a 6-month-old infant was dressed in girl's clothes and handed to a group of mothers, none of whom was the mother of this infant.[12] The infant was then dressed in boy's clothes and returned to the same group of mothers. The mothers responded differently to the "boy" than to the "girl" and described "him" as "different" from "her."

Studies of older children confirm the differences in rearing and indicate that many more subtle socialization pressures are operating. The responses to aggression, for example, constitute an important area, and girls are clearly taught to deal with aggression indirectly. There is at present no clear evidence to indicate that there are innate sex differences in the amount of aggression, although some authors feel there might be, but there is support for the hypothesis that males behave more aggressively than females.[45] It is apparent that parental behavior and the behavior of other important people have an enormous and early impact on children, and that studies of older children and adults that assess sex differences are reaching individuals who have already lived through years of differentiated experiences. This knowledge contributes to the greater emphasis in recent theory on the importance of object relations and real experience in contrast to the earlier, more exclusive focus on the development of the drives.

The importance of learning in these early years, based on the maturation of cognitive capacities, has been stressed recently.[3,46] Early psychoanalytic theorists did not really integrate it into their formulations. Learning includes the importance of language development and the concomitant categorizations that become possible when words exist.

I have mentioned the body image representation that divides girls and boys at an early age, and I have noted that observations support the view that young children have differentiated relationships to each parent, male and female. From their studies of preschool children, Galenson and Roiphe observed that castration anxieties appear earlier than were described by Freud.[46] These concerns are observed by the second half of the second year. They become apparent at the time that the child develops anxiety and fears of losing the people who are important to him or her. These fears are felt as possible dangers to the self because of the child's still-unstable sense of differentiation of the self and others. Castration fears are strongly influenced by the child's life experience, such as the nature of her or his relationships, their constancy, and the amount of stability or real loss that has occurred in the child's life.

In contrast to the early speculations about masturbation in little girls, data from clinical and research observations support the early awareness of the vagina in girls and confirm that girls' masturbation sometimes involves vaginal fantasies and play, so that the vagina forms part of the self-image.[30,47] The confusion many girls feel about their genitals is based partly on their hidden location and the taboos about examining them. This confusion is added to by parental mislabeling, in which the term *vagina* is used to refer to the female genitals as a whole, without a differentiation of labia, vulva, vagina, uterus, etc.[48] Since the little girl cannot actually see the organ she is told about, she is unable to confirm or clarify her fantasies and concepts.[48,49]

PENIS ENVY

The central position assigned to conflicts from the Oedipal stage and to penis envy as a stimulus to feminine development has shifted. Penis envy is no longer seen by most analysts as occupying as pivotal a position in women's psychological organization as was generally thought. It certainly exists as a concern for many women, consciously or unconsciously; but in adult women, if it is a major problem, it is generally in connection with other conflicts in which early deprivation, intense envy, and separations are important components. For other women, it is an issue that may be present to various degrees but is not the critical determinant of feminine development. Identity and self-esteem are seen from a broader perspective, and the origins of problems of self-esteem are not thought to be necessarily related to a sense of defectiveness because of anatomical inferiority. In fact, the degree of penis envy that Freud considered normal and necessary in order for the girl to achieve femininity is considered depressive by Clower,[30] and an indication of pathological envy or the incomplete resolution of separation–individuation. That is to say, the woman does not feel "whole" on her own.

In classical theory, the penis was thought to be valued for a variety of reasons: because it gave the little boy a special advantage in urination and showing off; because of its "fanciness"; because of the greater availability as a source of sexual pleasure and masturbation; and also as a symbol of status and power, which have been greater for men. One might, however, take a somewhat different position and question the girl's concern with her weakness, powerlessness, and devalued state, in which she sees herself as in need of some source of strength and specialness outside herself; as a result, she may regard the penis as this potential source of strength, without which she feels inadequate. A clinical vignette gives an illustration:

> A child analyst was treating a little girl with nightmares. To comfort herself and create a feeling of protection, she slept with a stuffed snake. The interpretation that this snake was a penis symbol that made her feel more powerful, like her father and brothers, may have been obvious. A therapist currently might, however, address himself or herself to the little girl's sense of vulnerability and defectiveness without this symbolic object and might understand this as the primary problem.

PASSIVITY

Passivity as a description of a central component of adult femininity is inaccurate and incomplete, since it does not address autonomous, assertive, individuated development in women. It is perhaps less valid as a description of most women than it once was. Yet, most women do feel conflicted about assertion and so do not easily use what abilities and talents they have. The changing of social patterns of what is acceptable does not automatically resolve these conflicts, and they persist clinically, although many women now are aware of them and wish to change. [10]

SELF-ESTEEM

Recent psychoanalytic development has involved considerable attention to "self-psychology" in Kohut's terms and to the "awareness of self" and self-esteem. [50] Self-esteem is difficult to define precisely but is an ego state involving an assessment of how one measures up to one's ego ideal; that is, the internalized values, goals, and standards of parents and others, which are also an indication of how one wants to be.

Self-esteem is defined by Jacobson as the "ideational, especially the emotional expression of self evaluation." [51] Self-esteem fluctuates within certain limits, depending on the responses of others and on one's own feeling of accomplishment, mastery, and value in a variety of areas.

Gender identity is inseparable from issues of self-esteem. An individual can feel good about herself if she feels adequate "as a woman," whatever the definition of that may be. *Unfeminine* is usually a term of criticism. Physical and sexual experiences and gratifications, as well as the acceptance of one's body and all its functions, were stressed by Thompson as basic to the establishment of self-respect and self-esteem. Women have found it difficult to acquire ease and pleasure from their bodies and their body image, and also to experience gratification and pleasure from the sensations emanating from their bodies.[3,29] They have often felt self-critical and depreciated, an experience that does not contribute to feeling good about oneself. The self-image of being "castrated" certainly lowers self-esteem. It implies that one is not whole or perfect or even as one "should be."

Kohut (1971) stated that "Self-esteem derives from a stable system of firmly idealized values"[50] and that under favorable circumstances, such as appropriate selective parental responses to the child's demands and to the manifestations of the child's grandiose fantasies, the child learns to accept his or her realistic limitations and grandiose fantasies; then, the crude, immature, exhibitionistic demands are given up and replaced by ego syntonic goals and purposes, by pleasure in his or her functions and activities, and by realistic self-esteem.

Therefore, major influences in the development of self-esteem are the attitudes of parents and identification with them, as well as "original narcissism," used here in a positive sense. In 1934, George Mead stated a similar view, namely, that the child "has achieved something of a self-concept through reacting to and internalizing the attitudes of family members to him."[52] He felt that self-esteem is gradually modified by experiences with peers and others but that the basic link to the parents is critical. Bibring wrote of the achievement of mastery that also leads to self-esteem by diminishing helplessness.[53] Jacobson regards self-esteem as being modulated by the superego and modified in response to actual experience. It is more fluctuating when unconscious conflicts exist. She believes that the child gradually moves away from the wish to be symbiotically tied to the parent (during the process described by Mahler as separation–individuation[26]) and toward acquiring the attributes of the parent and selectively identifying with that parent.[51]

Since the child needs and depends on parental love and approval and desires to live up to parental expectations, which are gradually internalized, the state of parental self-esteem and the parents' self-image is extremely important. For a woman whose mother felt devalued, which is true of many women, the struggle to achieve her own self-esteem may mean some psychic separation from and even rejection of the mother. Usually, this is not a conscious process but an unconscious one and may be manifested in a sense of distance, or hostility. The adolescent developmental goals of self-actualization and achievement of independence may also represent, in part, an attempt to separate from the devalued self-image of the mother.

Depression is a widespread problem for women. Weisman described the implications of maternal depression for children.[54,55] As mentioned earlier, the woman whose mother was depressed is likely to have problems with her own self-esteem unless other identification models have been available and she has had the capacity to make use of these new relationships and experiences. Many women who have depressed mothers do not develop the resources necessary for ego autonomy and may have difficulty working through self-esteem problems.

A discussion of self-esteem must also involve some consideration of aggression. As indicated earlier, women have not been permitted the direct expression of aggression or assertion that men have been allowed without feeling guilty or unfeminine.[49] Kaplan spoke of the inhibition of aggressive impulses in latency girls.[56] She described these impulses as self-directed, or followed by guilt if they are directed against others. Aggression used in this context refers not only to hostility, competitiveness, or destructive impulses and acts, but also to the assertiveness and free expression sometimes labeled *self-actualization*. To the extent that mastery, competence, the pursuit of personal goals, or competitive activity requires the recognition and expression of aggression or its derivatives, this awareness of being aggressive is likely to diminish self-esteem, and the woman feels a sense of worthlessness or wrongdoing.[49] This feeling can lead to conflicts for her because of the contradictions between the assertiveness required in work or other situations and internalized prohibitions. Contemporary views of women do acknowledge the importance of self-actualization, and there has been an increased acceptance of women's assertiveness and aggression as appropriate. This acceptance has taken the form of increased tolerance or even support for competitiveness in sports, in professional or business pursuits, and in other areas—some feel at the cost of more "human" feminine values. The balance has been difficult to achieve. Women's anger is still feared, and the openly aggressive woman has difficulties; even if the anger is appropriate, it can inhibit her work and other functioning. Horner has described the "fear of success" in a population of bright, achieving female students who were inhibited and blocked in their achievements, particularly when working with male students, because they perceived that success would cost them the loss of their relationship with males and of the esteem of the people around them.[57] These young women were afraid that they would be seen as unfeminine. In fact, they may have been correct, since many of the male students at that time were uncomfortable with the female students whom they regarded as competitive.

Dependency has been supported and reinforced for women. The term *learned helplessness* describes this process.[58] Little girls are also kept closer to their mothers than are little boys; they are encouraged to seek support and are permitted to express dependency needs.[58] They have, in the past, grown up expecting that they will be cared for by men—financially, at least—although at the same time, they are the providers of nurturance. To function more autonomously and independently can therefore threaten a woman's sense of "femininity."

Masochism is now viewed differently than it has been in the past. A truly masochistic individual, whether male or female, is considered pathological. Blum stated that "masochism is a residue of unresolved infantile conflict and is neither essentially feminine nor a valuable component of mature female function and character. Though the female might be more predisposed to masochism, there is no evidence of particular female pleasure in pain."[28] It is important to distinguish between masochistic suffering as a goal in itself and tolerance of deprivation, of discomfort, or even of suffering for the sake of some other goal or ideal. For instance, the effort one makes in an athletic pursuit might be termed "masochistic suffering" in another context, such as a woman's tolerating the pain of childbearing. It has been considered "heroic" to bear the pain of athletic stress or injury, usually an experience more common to men.

Women do characteristically find fulfillment by doing things for others rather than by acting on goals important primarily to themselves. They support their husbands and live through their children, and many of the careers they enter are service-oriented. Thus, they may have given up the fulfillment of their own needs for the sake of the relationships that are central to their lives.[31] Insofar as relationships and concern about the needs of others are central, it might be argued that women fulfill important humanistic values. In this sense, surrendering one's own goals for some larger good must also be distinguished from masochism in its classical sense.

Erikson addressed himself to female personality development, although most of his work, as is true of most theorists, has been concerned with men.[59,60] His theories have integrated the individual's development with social practices, customs, and beliefs, and he sees an individual as having lived and adapted throughout to a particular societal context. He stressed the sex differences in child rearing in several cultures and connected these with the kind of men and women who developed in each culture. Data from studies of play in 12- and 13-year-old American children led him to focus on sex differences in spatial orientation, which he saw as analogous to anatomical differences. He spoke of the "inner space" of the woman, reflected in the emphasis on enclosure, protection, and receptivity in the constructions of girls, and the protrusion, activity, and projection in the productions of boys: the emptiness that remained a potential for women led to a potential for depression and despair. He commented on the greater skills of women in those areas that enhance their ability to respond to the needs of others. Although he was clearly aware of socialization in the development of these tendencies, he did not explicitly acknowledge this awareness in his formulation.[59] He presented the anatomical basis for this difference, and although it is described in positive terms, with a stress on the capacity for nurturance and the value of intimacy and cooperation, it has nevertheless provoked attack from feminists, who object to the biological determinism that has been used in the past to support inequality rather than to emphasize positive differences. Erikson formulated eight stages in normal development, with a focus on the ego qualities that emerge from each: [60]

I. Basic trust	V. Identity
II. Autonomy	VI. Intimacy
III. Initiative	VII. Generativity
IV. Industry	VIII. Ego integrity

His eight stages have been criticized as applying more accurately to the development of males, in whom, for instance, the stage of identity precedes the stage of intimacy. Women's identity has been connected by Erikson with the achievement of intimacy with another.[60] Because of the particular character of feminine development, in which relationships are highly important, Gilligan stated that one might regard intimacy and identity as "fused" and developing together.[5,61] Erikson has also been criticized for the persistent identification of women with being mothers and with achieving their "identity" primarily through motherhood.

THE SIGNIFICANCE OF REPRODUCTION

The role and importance of childbearing in feminine identity have always been assumed. A woman's expectation of being able to bear children has been considered critical in the development of gender identity, femininity, and self-esteem. Nevertheless, in spite of their importance for human survival and the fact that fertility has been worshiped and considered sacred throughout history, childbearing and caretaking functions have generally occupied a lower place in the scale of status and prestige in most societies. Recent social changes, which have diminished the emphasis on reproduction and have resulted in the emergence of other alternatives for women, have provoked questions about life choices, which were previously felt to be automatic, about the concerns of femininity and feminine identity that were formerly seen as fundamental and accepted.[62]

Psychoanalytic theory has contributed to our understanding of the individual significance of childbearing. However, this has not been a central area of exploration, and most early writers saw motivations for motherhood as deriving from other developmental experiences. Although female sexuality was a critical area of investigation for Freud, Kestenberg (1956)[20] pointed to the relative scarcity of references to maternal needs and motherhood.

A number of authors have addressed themselves to the question of feminine identity and have attempted to create a concept of femininity based on standards of female rather than male development. However, as indicated earlier, there is no consistent agreement about the meaning of femininity nor the role of reproduction. More recent data from clinical observations, particularly in the past 10–15 years, not only support the early awareness of the vagina in girls but also contrast with Freud's view that the vagina was not important in itself.[28,46,63] Margaret Mead said, in criticism of Freud, that the vagina was not seen by him as "an entry into the womb but merely as a displacement from the clitoris."[64] Mead spoke for many critics in her view that the denigration of the value of producing a baby and the high valuation of the penis by both sexes were a fallacy of Freud's theories. This position was supported by others as well, writing prior to the current interest in female psychology.

Contemporary psychoanalytic thinking has also addressed the role of childbearing and child rearing in feminine identity particularly in the context of the major current changes in family patterns and the dramatic decline in the birth rate. Many children do not have the opportunity to observe pregnant women at close range, including their own mothers pregnant with younger siblings. Many young adult women are in conflict about a decision that used to be assumed, namely, that they would marry and have children. Femininity, for them, and fulfillment as a woman seem to require some revisions of self-image. Nevertheless, it seems likely that the capacity to bear children is significant, whether or not it is acted on as an adult choice. It is important to know that one's body can "work right."

In the construction of an understanding of women's psychology based on the study of female development and experience, the special anatomical aspects of the female body and the implications of her being the bearer of children are certainly critical. With the widening of roles

and responsibilities for women, reproductive potential and its defining role need reassessment. It is also important not to ignore the psychology of men and their changing roles and patterns in understanding female psychology.

More recently, not only motherhood but parenthood has been seen
as providing the experience of maturation for both men and women. [65]
The potential for the woman's growth through motherhood has been
stressed more consistently. For example, Benedek (1970) explicitly stated
that "Women have a better chance to achieve completion of their
physical and emotional maturation through motherhood than they have
if motherhood is denied to them." [65] Bibring saw pregnancy as a developmental crisis with maturational potential. [66] In her view, the gratifying experience of successful mothering established self-confidence.
Later, Benedek spoke of parenthood as a developmental phase, with
genuine ego maturation in both parents being a response to all levels
of the child's growth. Erikson emphasized "generativity" as a later
stage to be achieved in adult development. [60]

SUPEREGO DEVELOPMENT

Freud's observations on women's "sense of justice" and morality
are well known. He believed that women had little sense of justice
because of the predominance of envy in their mental life. [9] Freud was
not stating that men's morality was actually better than women's, but
this implication emerges from his descriptions. He said that

> For women the level of what is ethically moral is different from what it is
> in men. Their superego is never so inexorable, so impersonal, so indepen-
> dent of its emotional origins as we require it to be in men . . . they are
> less ready to submit to the great exigencies of life . . . they are more often
> influenced in their judgments by feelings of affection or hostility . . . all
> these would be amply accounted for in the modification of the formation
> of their superego. [16]

He regarded women's responsiveness to the emotional demands of the
people close to them as a potential corruption of an abstract sense of
fairness and justice.

The idea that moral reasoning and a sense of justice are best expressed by an adherence to abstract principles is also expressed in the
formulations of Kohlberg, who has developed a means of measuring
moral development in which the highest stage is the most principled
and abstract. Gilligan has criticized this approach as reflecting primarily male development and style. [5]

In a critique of Freud's psychology of women, Schafer referred to
the quality of moral rigidity that he finds characterizes men more than

women.[67] Schafer stated that Freud was referring to the greater capacity for isolation of affect that is true of many men, and he stressed that the greater predominance of obsessive morality is founded on reaction formation against sadistic, aggressive tendencies and intense unconscious guilt and is therefore a poor model of morality. He further argued against the appropriateness of morality detached from the fear of loss of love, a characteristic of women that Freud described and thought of as a source of potential weakness. It is paradoxical to note that it is a widely held belief that women are the "guardians of civilized conduct and morality." Many have also thought that it is more important in the long run, for the survival of humanity, to have a less abstract and a more responsive justice, although retaining objectivity and fairness. Schafer also emphasized the intrusion of patriarchal and evolutionary values into Freud's judgments, in which observed qualitative differences are referred to as differences in worth or maturity.

There are wide variations in superego development between individuals. However, those differences that may be characteristic of women as compared with men can be seen in the light of their complex antecedents and functions, and not merely as reflecting "better" or "worse" styles.

IMPLICATIONS FOR TREATMENT

A fuller discussion of the implications for therapy is found in Volume 3 of this series. It is important to emphasize here that although many would assert that a "good" therapist or psychoanalyst has his or her patients' goals in mind rather than intruding his or her own values, in practice this is not always the case, and judgments are consciously or unconsciously influenced by one's own point of view.[68] Some authors have stressed the importance of the recognition that therapists do indeed have values and often represent societal positions. "Feminist therapists" have also asserted that it is important for a patient to know the therapist's values. While such knowledge may have some advantages, it is extremely difficult to acquire and can also provide diversion from the central therapeutic goals.

In some areas, therapeutic norms and practices have been influenced by changes in thinking about women. The expansion of what is viewed as a "normal" or "feminine" life pattern has been considerable. Attention to the unconscious interference and conflicts of the past and the resolution of current issues is not necessarily different from the concerns of therapy in the past, but assumptions about appropriate resolutions may have shifted.

Women are not expected to spend their entire time at home or with their children, even when their children are small. In most settings, the mother is regarded as—and, in fact, is—the primary caretaker, so there is still great emphasis in theory on "mother–child" interactions, but there is also an increasing acknowledgment of the role of family factors and of the importance of the father in the development of the child. This shift has contributed to changes in what are thought to be the appropriate concerns and activities of a "masculine" person as well as a "feminine" one.

Goals for women include their own wishes for self-actualization as well as their reproductive goals. Most women do want to marry and have children, but this is not assumed to be the only appropriate goal, nor is a treatment judged successful if its primary accomplishment is, like the resolutions in the fairy tales, that the woman marries and lives happily ever after. Work is recognized as an important part of women's lives. Thus, therapists are reflecting the major societal shift of women's entering the work force in rapidly increasing numbers. There have been changes in the expectation of marital roles and styles, and therapists need to approach problems of new lifestyles with openness and understanding.[69]

Transference issues remain central to psychoanalytic psychotherapy. However, it is important to differentiate a patient's bringing to her treatment the expectations, fantasies, and responses to her therapist that arise from childhood relationships and need to be explored and understood before she can function freely as an adult, from the authority aspects of the doctor–patient or therapist–patient relationship, which are assumed to be a part of the appropriate social interaction between a male therapist and female patient and are therefore not analyzed or explored. In many ways, psychotherapy for women reflects the changing issues in psychotherapy for all patients and will continue to respond to societal changes, at the same time continuing to include the goals of relief of pain and suffering and improvement in the capacity for attaining fulfillment and creativity.

REFERENCES

1. Horney K: The flight from womanhood, *International Journal of Psychoanalysis* 7:324–339, 1926. Reprinted in *Psychoanalysis and women.* Edited by Miller J. New York, Brunner/Mazel, 1973.
2. Jones E: Early female sexuality, *International Journal of Psychoanalysis* 6:263–273, 1935.
3. Thompson C: Some effects of the derogatory attitude towards female sexuality, *Psychiatry* 13:349–354, 1980.
4. Zilboorg G: Masculine and feminine: Some biological and cultural aspects, *Psychiatry* 7:257–296, 1944.
5. Gilligan C: In a different voice: Women's conception of the self and morality, *Harvard Educational Review* 47 (4):481–517, 1977.

6. Sherman J: *On the psychology of women.* Springfield, Ill., Charles C Thomas, 1971.
7. Chasseguet-Smirgel J: Feminine guilt and the Oedipus complex, in *Female sexuality.* Edited by Chasseguet-Smirgel J. Ann Arbor, University of Michigan Press, pp. 94–134, 1970.
8. Chasseguet-Smirgel J: "Introduction," in *Female sexuality.* Edited by Chasseguet-Smirgel J. Ann Arbor, Univeristy of Michigan Press, pp. 1–3, 1970.
9. Freud S (1933): Femininity, new introductory lectures, in *Standard edition of the complete works of Sigmund Freud.* Edited by Strachey J. London: Hogarth Press, 1961.
10. Notman M, Nadelson C, Bennet M: Achievement conflict in women: Psychotherapeutic considerations, *Psychotherapy and Psychosomatic* 29:203–213, 1978.
11. Moss HA: Sex, age and state as determinants of mother-infant interaction, *Merrill-Palmer Quarterly* 13:19–36, 1967.
12. Will J, Self P, Datan N: Maternal behavior and perceived sex of infants, *American Journal of Orthopsychiatry* 46 (1):135–139, 1976.
13. Maccoby E, Jacklin E: *The psychology of sex differences.* Stanford, Calif., Stanford University Press, 1974.
14. Parsons J, Ruble D: Is anatomy destiny? Biology and sex differences, in *Women and sex roles.* Edited by Frieze I, et al. New York: Norton, 1978.
15. Deutsch H: *The psychology of women.* Vols. 1, 2. New York: Grune & Stratton, 1944, 1945.
16. Freud S: Femininity, new introductory lectures, in *Standard edition of the complete psychological works of Sigmund Freud,* Vol. 19. Edited by Strachey J. London, Hogarth Press, 1961.
17. Freud S (1925): Some psychical consequences of the anatomical distinction between the sexes, in *Standard edition of the complete psychological works of Sigmund Freud,* Vol. 19. Edited by Strachey J. London, Hogarth Press, 1961.
18. Freud S (1931): Female sexuality, in Introductory Lectures, in *Standard edition of the complete psychological works of Sigmund Freud,* Vol. 21. Edited by Strachey J. London, Hogarth Press, 1961.
19. Klein M: *Early stages in the Oedipal conflict in the psychoanalysis of children.* New York, Grove Press, 1962.
20. Kestenberg J: Vicissitudes of female sexuality, *Journal of American Psychoanalytic Association* 4:453–475, 1956. Revised and republished in Kestenberg J: *Children and parents.* New York, Aronson, 1975.
21. Benedek T: *Psychosexual functions in women.* New York, Ronald Press, 1952.
22. Bonaparte M: *Female sexuality.* New York, International University Press, 1953.
23. Benedek T: The psychology of pregnancy, in *Parenthood.* Edited by Anthony J, Benedek T. Boston, Little, Brown, p. 139, 1970.
24. Winnicot D: The mother-infant experience of mutuality, in *Parenthood.* Edited by Anthony J, Benedek T. Boston, Little, Brown, pp. 246–255, 1970.
25. Brazelton T: *Infants and mothers.* New York, Delacorte Press, 1969.
26. Mahler M, Pine F, Bergman A: *The psychological birth of the human infant.* New York, Basic Books, 1975.
27. Freud S: The economic problem of masochism, in *Standard edition of the complete psychological works of Sigmund Freud,* Vol. 19. Edited by Strachey J. London: Hogarth Press, pp. 157–170, 1961.
28. Blum H: Masochism, the ego ideal and the psychology of women, *Journal of the American Psychoanalytic Association* 24 (5):157–191, 1976.
29. Easser R: *Womanhood.* Unpublished manuscript, prepared for the Panel on Female Psychology, American Psychoanalytic Association, 1975.
30. Clower V: Theoretical implications of current views of masturbation in latency girls, *Journal of the American Psychoanalytic Association* 24 (5):109–125, 1976.

31. Miller J: *Towards a new psychology of women*. Boston, Beacon Press, 1976.
32. Ruble D: Sex differences in personality and abilities, in *Women and sex roles: A social psychological perspective*. Edited by Frieze I, *et al*. New York: Norton, pp. 45–68, 1978.
33. Stoller R: Overview, the impact of new advances in sex research on psychoanalytic theory, *American Journal of Psychiatry* 132:241–251, 1973.
34. Stoller R: Primary femininity, *Journal of the American Psychoanalytic Association 24* (5):59–78, 1976.
35. Money J, Enhardt A: *Man and woman, boy and girl*. Baltimore, Johns Hopkins Press, 1972.
36. Abelin E: Some further observations and comments on the earliest role of the father, *International Journal of Psychoanalysis 56*:293–302, 1975.
37. Hoffman L, Nye F: *Working mothers*. San Francisco, Jossey-Bass, 1974.
38. Galenson E: Report of panel on early infancy and childhood, *Journal of the American Psychoanalytic Association 24* (1):141–160, 1976.
39. Riviere J: On the genesis of psychical conflicts in early infancy, *International Journal of Psychoanalysis 17*:395–422, 1937.
40. Brunswick R: The pre-Oedipal phase of the libido development, *Psychoanalytic Quarterly 9*:293–319, 1940.
41. Lampl de Groot L: Problems of femininity, *Psychoanalytic Quarterly 2*:489–518, 1933.
42. Chodorow N: *The reproduction of mothering: Psychoanalysis and the sociology of gender*. Berkeley, University of California Press, 1978.
43. Rossi A: A biosocial perspective on parenting, *Daedalus*, pp. 1–31, Spring 1977.
44. Moss R: Sex, age and state as determinants of mother-infant interaction, in *Reading in the psychology of women*. Edited by Brunswick J. New York: Harper & Row, pp. 22–29, 1972.
45. Rubler D: Sex differences in personality and abilities, in *Women and sex roles*. Edited by Frieze I, *et al*. New York, Norton, p. 54, 1978.
46. Galenson E, Roiphe H: Some suggested revisions concerning early female development, *Journal of the American Psychoanalytic Association 24* (5):29–57, 1976.
47. Williams J: *The emergence of sex differences in psychology of women*. New York, Norton, pp. 121–157, 1977.
48. Lerner H: Parental mislabelling of female genitals as a determinant of penis envy and learning inhibitions in women, *Journal of the American Psychoanalytic Association 24* (5):269–283, 1976.
49. Zilbach J, Notman M, Nadelson C, Miller J: *Reconsideration of aggression and self-esteem in women*. Presentation at the International Psychoanalytic Association, New York, August 1, 1979.
50. Kohut H: *The analysis of self*. New York, International Universities Press, 1971.
51. Jacobson E: The regulation of self-esteem, in *Depression and human existence*. Edited by Anthony EJ, Benedet T. Boston, Little, Brown, 1975.
52. Mead G: *Mind, self and society*. Chicago, University of Chicago Press, 1934.
53. Bibring G: The mechanism of depression in affective disorders, in *Affective disorders*. Edited by Greenacre P. New York: International Universities Press, pp. 13–48, 1953.
54. Weissman M, Paykel E: *The depressed woman*. Chicago, University of Chicago Press, 1974.
55. Weissman M, Klerman G: Sex differences and the epidemiology of depression, *Archives of General Psychiatry 34*:98–111, 1977.
56. Kaplan E: Manifestations of aggression in latency and pre-adolescent girls, *Psychoanalytic Study of the Child 31*:63–78, 1976.
57. Horner M: Toward an understanding of achievement-related conflicts in women, *Journal of Social Issues 28*:157–175, 1972.

58. Gove W: Sex differences in the epidemiology of mental disorder: Evidence and explanations, in *Gender and disordered behavior*. Edited by Gromberg E, Franks V. New York, Brunner/Mazel, pp. 23–68, 1979.
59. Erikson E: Womanhood and the inner space, in *Identity, youth and crisis*. Edited by Erikson E. New York, Norton, pp. 261–294, 1968.
60. Erikson E: *Childhood and society*. New York, Norton, 1950.
61. Gilligan C: Women's place in man's life cycle, *Harvard Educational Review 49* (4):431–446, 1979.
62. Notman M, Nadelson C: *New views of femininity and reproduction*. Presented at the Annual Meeting of the American Psychiatric Association, Chicago, May 1978.
63. Kleeman J: Freud's views on early female sexuality in the light of direct child observation, *Journal of the American Psychoanalytic Association 24* (5):3–27, 1976.
64. Mead M: *Male and female*. New York, William Morrow, 1949.
65. Benedek T: Parenthood as a developmental phase, in *Parenthood: Its psychology and psychopathology*. Edited by Anthony J, Benedek T. Boston, Little, Brown, 1970.
66. Bibring G: Some considerations of the psychological process in pregnancy, *The Psychoanalytic Study of the Child 14*:113–121, New York, International Universities Press, 1959.
67. Schafer R: Problems in Freud's psychology of women. *Journal of the American Psychoanalytic Association 22*:459–485, 1974.
68. Broverman I, Broverman D, *et al*: Sex role stereotypes and clinical judgements of mental health, *Journal of Consulting and Clinical Psychology 34*:1–7, 1970.
69. Franks V: Gender and Psychotherapy, in *Gender and disordered behavior*. Edited by Gomberg E, Franks V. New York, Brunner/Mazel, pp. 453–485, 1979.

Chapter 2

Changing Views of the Relationship between Femininity and Reproduction

MALKAH NOTMAN AND CAROL NADELSON

There are substantial differences in the lifestyles of women today as compared with a generation ago. Fewer women are viewing marriage and motherhood as the central goals of their entire lives. Many are marrying later and having fewer or no children. In light of these changes, it seems appropriate to reexamine some concepts about femininity and feminine identity, as well as their relationship to reproduction.

For a woman, the knowledge that she is able to bear children has always been considered critical to the development of gender identity, femininity, and self-esteem. The emergence of acceptable, widely chosen alternative ways for women to order their lives has provoked questions about life choices that were previously felt to be automatic and has challenged concepts of femininity and feminine identity that were formerly seen as fundamental and immutable.

How is one to evaluate and understand feminine development and identity, as separate from childbearing? What are the implications for those women who do not actually have children? Does this lack of children inevitably mean a sense of failure and a lack of fulfillment for them? Are those women who are choosing not to have children expressing conflict about femininity and an incomplete realization of their feminine potential?

MALKAH NOTMAN, M.D. AND CAROL NADELSON, M.D. ● Department of Psychiatry, Tufts University School of Medicine-New England Medical Center Hospital, Boston, Massachusetts¹.

Unlimited fecundity has also come to be seen as less adaptive in the face of population expansion and the development of reasonably effective conception controls.[1] The birthrate in Western industrialized countries has dropped at the same time that better medical care has increased neonatal survival.

The uniqueness of women as the sole caretakers of their children has, in many instances, diminished, as mothers have increasingly shared "mothering" with fathers and others. Researchers have stressed the value, for the development of both children and fathers, of having fathers involved not only in the support of the mother and in relating to older children, but also in nurturing young infants.[2,3,4,5] Fathers themselves have also desired more active and meaningful participation in the lives of their children. Family structure and dynamics have also been affected by shifts in the definitions of sex roles that blur some of the distinctions between feminine and masculine roles and activities.[6]

THEORETICAL ISSUES

Psychoanalytic theory has contributed to our understanding of the significance of childbearing to the individual. However, this has not been a central area of psychoanalytic exploration, and most earlier psychoanalysts saw motivations for motherhood as deriving from other developmental experiences. Although female sexuality was a critical area of investigation for Freud, Kestenberg pointed to the relative scarity of references to maternal needs and motherhood.[7] Freud thought of the female psyche as enigmatic. He felt that girls and boys developed similarly for the first three years and considered the little girl "masculine" until the development of femininity, when she felt disappointed in her mother, who had failed to give her a penis, and turned to her father, with an unconscious wish for a baby. Freud saw two sources for the wish for a baby, one associated with a passive feminine attitude, which he termed the "anal baby," and one derived from the "active masculinity" of the phallic phase, the "penis baby." He theorized that the original wish for a penis was replaced by a wish for a child. Freud, Deutsch, and others viewed the responses of a woman as a mother as "active" in contrast to the overall passivity of femininity, but they described it as "appropriate" activity.[8,9] There was some confusion between this kind of activity and the activity characterizing "masculinity"; and the activity of motherhood was at times considered "sublimated masculinity," or "substitutive masculinity," or some other aspect of masculinity.[10]

In searching for the sources of motherliness, Deutsch also thought a baby was perceived as a substitute for the woman's lack of a penis. She found it difficult to decide to what extent motherliness was biologically determined. Kestenberg described the development of maternal feelings as an integral part of the development of female sexuality.[11] She viewed the source of motherly feelings as arising from the sensations and libido derived from the vagina and from the little girl's awareness of this part of her body. She described an "inner genital phase."[11]

Benedek also searched for the biological roots of the feelings associated with pregnancy and motherhood, and she saw the major basis for these in the fluctuation of the female endocrine cycle.[12] She studied this cycle and concluded that the "deep rooted passivity" and "tendency toward introversion," described by Deutsch, were characteristic of the female psyche and that they appeared mostly in connection with the postovulative phase of the menstrual cycle.[13] She concluded further that "the emotional manifestations of the specific receptive tendency and the self-centered retentive tendency are the psychodynamic correlates of a biologic need for motherhood," and therefore that motherhood is not secondary or a substitute for the missing penis, nor is it forced by men upon women "in the service of the species"; rather, it is the manifestation of an "instinct for survival in the child that is the primary organizer of the women's sexual drive and her personality."[13]

In this attitude, Benedek anticipated current writers who stress the nonsubstitutive nature of the wish for a child, and who describe the reciprocal nature of the development of motherly feelings as a response to the infant's needs. Although developmental identification with one's mother was seen by Benedek and others as an important determinant of a woman's emotional attitude toward motherhood and of her mothering behavior, the central role of the early identification with the mother was not emphasized as much by these writers as were the biological, or instinctual, origins of mothering behavior and of female drive organization.[14] Adult women's psychological attitudes were thought to be dependent on hormonal or other biological factors, and the idea of the wish for a baby as a replacement for the organ she did not have was prevalent in the literature.

Feminine development was also conceptualized in relation to the question of whether early vaginal sensations existed, and whether the little girl was aware of the vagina or of other organs that could contain a baby. Those who felt that the little girl did have some awareness of the vagina assumed the earlier development of "femininity."[15,16] Those who supported the concept of the "initial masculinity" of the little girls, which was the view held by Freud, felt that the vagina was dis-

covered only at puberty and that "true" femininity developed only
then.[9,10] They thought that the little girl's early body image was that
she had a "small penis" (i.e., the clitoris), which was the source of
her disappointment with herself and her mother for having "made
her" that way.

More recently, writers have challenged the view of the woman as
anatomically defective because of the absence of a penis, as well as the
functions of childbearing as a substitute for this absence.[17,18,19] They
have also emphasized again, as did Horney and Thompson earlier,
that childbearing has its origin in positive feminine identity as well.[15,20]

A number of authors have addressed themselves to the question
of feminine identity and its endogenous sources and childhood manifestations. They have attempted to create a concept of femininity based
on standards of female rather than male development. However, the
component elements of femininity are not uniformly agreed on, nor is
the role of reproduction. More recent data from clinical observations,
particularly in the past 10–15 years, support the early awareness of the
vagina in girls and also challenge Freud's view that the vagina is not
important in itself.[17,18,21] Margaret Mead presented this point of view
when she criticized Freud for thinking of the vagina not as the entry
into the womb, and thus an important part of the woman's genital
and reproductive organs, but as a displacement from the clitoris.[22]

Direct observations of children and of the process of gender identity formation, as distinguished from the consideration of sexual fantasies and behavior, indicate that earlier ideas that were based on reconstructions from work with adults were erroneous. Stoller has
proposed the term "primary femininity" to describe the first stage in
female development.[18] This involves the establishment of a sense of
being rightfully a female, based on the combinations of biological factors, sex assignment at birth, parental attitudes, early postnatal effects
caused by conditioning, and developing body sensations, especially
from the genitals. He feels that this is a nonconflictual stage. The second stage of feminine development, he postulated, does result from
conflict, particularly Oedipal conflict (see Chapter 1).

Nevertheless, an important component of femininity in most formulations includes a central position for pregnancy and motherhood.
The importance of the pre-Oedipal identification with the mother and
of the cognitive processes that are important in the development of
early gender identity (that is, learning what "goes with" being female)
and the awareness of "feminine" style, as it is expressed in a given
culture, has been emphasized recently. This awareness also includes
the expectation of having children, or at least an awareness of one's

biological capacity to have them, whether or not this capacity is ful-filled for a given individual.[9,13,23,24]

Parenthood, not only motherhood, has also been seen as provid-ing experience for maturation.[23,25] Although this view includes both parents, the potential for women's growth through motherhood was stressed earlier and has been emphasized more consistently. For ex-ample, Benedek explicitly stated in 1952, "Women have a better chance to achieve completion of their physical and emotional maturation through motherhood than they have if motherhood is denied to them." Bibring also saw pregnancy as a potentially maturational developmen-tal crisis for the mother.[26] Old identifications were "loosened" by a new potential for growth, and the rewarding experience of successful mothering established self-confidence. Benedek spoke of *parenthood* as a developmental phase and of genuine maturation in the parent as a potential response to the child's growth.[14] Erikson spoke of "genera-tivity," which is related to the care of the next generation, as a later stage to be achieved in adult development. It was, in fact, in regard to parenting that he first paid attention to the continued psychological development of the individual throughout adulthood.

BIOLOGICAL DETERMINANTS

The biological basis of pregnancy does not have to be seen as implying a unique and sufficient source for maternalism and nurtur-ance, although it provides a basis for women to start the experience of nurturance earlier and more intimately than men. Recent research in-volving the role of hormones and behavior suggests that the biological correlates are important. Several authors, using empirical and cross-cultural data, have emphasized this point.[27,28] They have also sug-gested that women's nurturance comes not only from biology, sociali-zation, and expectations, but from exposure to newborns as well. Fur-ther support for this view derives from data on mother–infant separation and its effects and from mother–infant bonding.[29,30,31] The vast literature on mothering demonstrates that what is required is not simply a set of behaviors, but participation in an important affective relationship, and these abilities are embedded in one's personality and emotional capacities (see Chapter 5).

DIVERGENT VIEWS ABOUT REPRODUCTION

It is interesting to look at the range of recent divergent positions about reproduction, perhaps expressing the different components of "what women want," a question Freud raised. Many feminists have stressed the need for better care for pregnant women. They have promoted more sensitive, humane medical attitudes and behavior, and also the allowing of more control of childbearing by the woman rather than by the medical profession. Caution about, and even suspicion of, the medical establishment and about procedures and medications has been advocated in the context of supporting childbearing.[32] Thus, safe, supported, optimally cared-for reproduction continues to be a central part of women's concerns.

At the same time, there has been a strong advocacy of freedom of choice about pregnancy, such as providing available and safe abortions. This dichotomy is not new. Deutsch, a proponent of the central role of motherhood in women's lives, also supported freedom of choice about childbearing and abortion.[9]

Additional evidence of the continued focus on the importance of reproductive choice, as well as alternatives to traditional childbearing patterns, is found in other cultural changes. The participation of fathers from the beginning of pregnancy—including prenatal care, labor, and delivery—and in early child care has been advocated. Another focus has been on creating more supports for working mothers, such as adequate day care. There has also been greater advocacy of the recognition of alternative lifestyles, such as lesbianism, singleness, an emphasis on work, a commitment to the fulfillment of career goals, and equality with men in work and career opportunities. These different ways of organizing one's life may or may not involve having children. The simplistic view that regards these alternatives as a denial of femininity is no longer viable.

The view that "conflicts about femininity" were the basis of psychosomatic gynecological disorders was based on a concept of feminine identity as defined by reproductive potential. This simplistic formulation has been replaced to some extent by a search for other mediating mechanisms of psychic conflict that might be expressed as organic pathology. Endocrine studies, EEGs, and a variety of psychological and other tests have been reported, and their connection with emotional problems has been explored; these studies have raised questions about traditional "understanding" as well as providing evidence that some obstetrical and gynecological problems do indeed reflect conflict about feminine functioning and about having a child, or ambivalence about a particular pregnancy.[33,34]

The data about the premenstrual syndrome and menopause are good examples of changes in views as information undermines earlier stereotyping. For example, careful studies of the menstrual cycle indicate that the symptoms reported vary if the subject is aware of the purpose of the study, and that behavioral measures show fewer differences than self-reported symptoms.[33] Similarly, careful attention to data about menopausal symptoms indicates that most symptomatology ascribed to the menopause is not related to actual menopausal status.[35,36] Nor is this ending of reproductive possibility inevitably associated with depression and feelings of loss or regret.[37]

To provide additional perspective on the relationship between childbearing and femininity, we examine here data on those who choose voluntary childlessness and those who are involuntarily infertile, and we also consider briefly those gynecological problems that have been understood as expressing conflicts about femininity.

VOLUNTARY CHILDLESSNESS

According to recent data, childlessness has increased (see Chapter 6). Estimates of the increase of voluntary childlessness based on an analysis of a variety of trends see it approaching 10%. Attitudes about having children have also changed. A number of recent studies show that the number of college women preferring childlessness increased; in one study, the increase was from 1% to 9% between 1961 and 1971.[38] Although the pendulum may be swinging back, the freedom of choice is unlikely to disappear.

Veevers has written an extensive review of the literature on childlessness.[39] She stressed the social pressure for having children, termed "pronatalism," and the negative attitudes toward those who elect childlessness, who are seen as physically blemished or "immoral." She described the "motherhood mandate" as a moral imperative for procreation and child care and stated that this imperative is especially emphatic for women and affects their concept of the female gender role. She cited the tendency to see those electing childlessness as demonstrating evidence of poor mental health and abnormality, or to see childlessness itself as leading to other atypical or deviant behavior or placing women at a disadvantage because they are deprived of a developmental opportunity for generativity, in Erikson's terms.

Childlessness is, however, not inevitably associated with distress. Its effects are complex, and other developmental opportunities may take the place of the experiences of childbearing and parenting.

A number of sociological studies indicate that smaller families are "happier" than larger ones, and that voluntarily childless couples are not unhappy.[40,41,42] For example, Campbell et al.'s extensive national survey concluded that the decision not to have children does not "doom the couple to loneliness and despair and misery."[40]

Veevers concluded, in summary, that the

> Available data do indicate that the consequences of remaining childless are
> somewhat different than the consequences of having children. Compared
> with parents, childless persons appear to have somewhat lower rates of
> morbidity. No systematic differences pertain with regards to mental health.
> For women, occupational success, especially exceptional success, seems to
> be significantly facilitated by remaining childless.[39]

Childlessness, whether voluntary or involuntary, certainly allows
more time for professional or other activities. An interesting observation from a study of those individuals listed in Who's Who indicates
that there are significant sex differences in childlessness in those
listed.[39] Among the women listed, rates of childlessness are much
higher than in the general population, although the proportion of
never-married childless women in this group declined from 54% in
1926 to 43% in 1948, and further, to 24% in 1979.[39,43] This shift may
indicate that there is some change in the view that marriage and children exclude major career commitments, as they did in the past. For
comparable men listed in Who's Who, the rates of childlessness were
generally slightly lower than in the general population. An observation consistent with this finding is that productivity as measured by
papers written is inversely related to the number of children men have.

The data from these studies concerning the motivation of childless
couples are generally not of sufficient depth to warrant definitive psychological conclusions. However, attitudes do emerge. Childless couples either discredit the worth and value of parental roles and experience or maximize or exaggerate these, with the implication that they
cannot be good parents. Some women have had reason to fear pregnancy or their competence as mothers, or having been first children in
large families, they feel unwilling to play that role again. Others prefer
the freedom of childlessness.

Preliminary studies of women who elect sterilizations indicate that
many of them base this decision on an assessment of their own capacities to mother and a history of difficulties with their own mothers,
and that they cannot necessarily be viewed as showing psychopathology or disturbance.[44] Ambivalence about mothering can now be more
easily expressed in one's life by not having children because of the
greater social tolerance of childlessness and other roles for women.

Clinically and demographically, it is apparent that many women
are waiting to have children until past the age that was considered
desirable a generation ago. Some of these women are establishing
themselves occupationally and financially first; others are changing their
minds and deciding to have a child as midlife approaches and possibilities begin to seem finite. For some, an important issue demanding
resolution is the separation from their own mothers and some confi-

dence that becoming a mother will not inevitably draw them back into the same lifestyle as their parents.

INVOLUNTARY STERILITY

Those who are involuntarily sterile have a different set of concerns.[45] The couple is confronted with a change in life plans and self-concept that can be very profound. The narcissistic injury, the loss of control over one's life, the mourning for what parenthood meant, and the readjustment of identity and redefining of femininity (for the man, masculinity) may be enormous and surprising, since neither partner, but particularly the woman, may have realized the personal importance of having a child.

It is difficult to separate the sense of defectiveness at having a body that does not function properly from the specific incapacity to have a child. Although infertility affects a man's confidence about his masculinity, the impact of this problem on the woman's sense of femininity is even greater, since the responsibility for having or not having children is still generally ascribed to the woman. Further, women continue to feel that it is their "fault" if they do not become pregnant, even when contradictory evidence is presented.[12,39] Not only are femininity and masculinity affected, but adult status is closely associated with parenthood, and the infertile couple may have a more difficult time negotiating the transition into adulthood with their own parents as well as with each other. This is where problems of "generativity" may become manifest.

The psychodynamics of infertility have been oversimplified in the past. The literature contains many references to the concept that infertility is a defense against the dangers that the individual, especially the woman, perceives as connected with procreation, and authors have written of the "repudiation of femininity" and of hostility to men as the causes of a variety of gynecological and emotional symptoms, including infertility, as well as of problems during pregnancy.[9,12,46] If a woman with this psychological constellation should by chance conceive, these problems were also thought to extend to parenting.[9]

As interesting as individual cases may be, empirical studies do not support a clear-cut emotional etiology of infertility in most cases.[47,48] Furthermore, even if the diagnosis of psychogenic infertility is made, the connection with "femininity" is unclear; in reality, it is far more complex. We do know that endocrine functioning is reciprocally influenced by psychological state, but direct causal relationships are difficult to define.[33,49] Anxiety about parenthood, adult roles, problem identifications with one's own parents, and anxiety about the adequate functioning of one's own body may inhibit proper sexual functioning, either by actual sexual dysfunction or by problems with ovulation, cervical secretions, or spasm of some part of the reproductive tract.[50,51]

CONCLUSION

We are left with more questions than answers. It seems clear that the individual and cultural meaning of reproduction is highly important to a given woman, and while the potential for childbearing is an important component of femininity, it is not entirely the central issue. A woman's self-esteem derives in part from this capacity, but other expressions of creativity are also important. The concept of femininity has undergone many changes, beginning with the descriptive triad of masochism, narcissism, and passivity, which have all been abandoned in their original versions as essential to normal feminine functioning. It seems that femininity itself (and masculinity as well) is a shifting and variable concept, intimately related to the woman's awareness of the capacity to bear and nurture children, but not invariably depending on this capacity for realization. Further clarification and a deeper understanding of the complex meanings of the fundamental distinctions between men and women in the formation of self-definition and self-esteem will depend on more careful observations and understanding of feminine development.

REFERENCES

1. U.S.Bureau of the Census: *Statistical Abstract of the United States*, 98th ed., pp. 6, 55, 1977.
2. Lynn D: *The father: His role in child development*. Monterey, Calif., Brooks/Cole, 1974.
3. Gurwitt A: Aspects of prospective fatherhood, *Psychoanalytic Study of the Child* 31:237–271, 1976.
4. Abelin E: Some further observations and comments on the earliest role of the father, *International Journal of Psychoanalysis* 56:293–302, 1975.
5. Lamb M: Fathers, *Human Development* 18:245–266, 1975.
6. Frieze I, Parsons J, Johnson P, et al.; *Women and sex roles*. New York, Norton, 1978.
7. Kestenberg J: On the development of maternal feelings in early childhood, *Psychoanalytic Study of the Child* 11:257–291, 1956.
8. Freud S (1925): Some psychical consequences of the anatomical distinction between the sexes. *Standard Edition*, Vol. 19, pp. 248–258. London, Hogarth Press, 1961.
9. Deutsch H: *The psychology of women. Motherhood*. Vol. 2. New York, Grune & Stratton, 1945.
10. Freud S: *Female sexuality. Collected papers*. London, Hogarth Press, 1950.
11. Kestenberg J: Vicissitudes of female sexuality. *Journal of the American Psychoanalytic Association* 4:453–476, 1956.

12. Benedek T: The psychosomatic implications of the primary unit: Mother-child, *American Journal of Orthopsychiatry* 19:642–654, 1949. Also in Benedek T, Rubenstein B: *Psychosexual functions in women*. New York, Ronald Press, 1952.

13. Benedek T: The psychobiology of pregnancy, in *Parenthood: Its psychology and psychopathology*. Edited by Anthony J, Benedek T. Boston: Little, Brown, pp. 137–151, 1970.

14. Benedek T: Mothering and nurturing, in *Parenthood: Its psychology and psychopathology*. Edited by Anthony E, Benedek T. Boston: Little, Brown, pp. 153–165, 1970.

15. Horney K: The flight from womanhood, *International Journal of Psychoanalysis* 7:324–339, 1926. Reprinted in Miller J: *Psychoanalysis and women*. New York, Brunner/Mazel, 1973.

16. Jones E: Early female sexuality, *International Journal of Psychoanalysis* 16:263–372, 1935.

17. Clower V: Theoretical implications on current views of masturbation in latency girls, *Journal of the American Psychoanalytic Association. Supplement: Female Psychology* 24 (5):109–125, 1976.

18. Stoller R: Primary femininity, *Journal of the American Psychoanalytic Association* 24 (5):59–78, 1976.

19. Chasseguet-Smirgel J: Feminine guilt and the Oedipus complex, in *Female sexuality*. Edited by Chasseguet-Smirgel J. Ann Arbor, University of Michigan, pp. 94–134, 1970.

20. Thompson C: Some effects of the derogatory attitude towards female sexuality, *Psychiatry* 13:349–354, 1950. Reprinted in Miller J: *Psychoanalysis and women*. New York, Brunner/Mazel, 1973.

21. Galenson E, Roiphe H: Some suggested revisions concerning early female development, *Journal of the American Psychoanalytic Association* 24 (5):29–57, 1976.

22. Mead M: *Male and female*. New York, William Morrow, 1949.

23. Erikson E: Identity and the Life Cycle: Selected papers, *Psychological Issues* 1:1–171, 1959.

24. Erikson E: Inner and outer space: Reflections on womanhood, *Daedalus* 93:582–608, 1964.

25. Benedek T: Infertility as a psychosomatic defense, *Fertility and Sterility* 3:527–537, 1952.

26. Bibring G: Some considerations of the psychological process of pregnancy, *Psychoanalytic Study of the Child* 14:13–121, 1959.

27. Maccoby E, Jacklin C: *The psychology of sex differences*. Stanford, Calif., Stanford University Press, pp. 214–221, 1974.

28. Chodorow N: *The reproduction of mothering, psychoanalysis and the sociology of gender*. Berkeley, University of California Press, 1978.

29. Klaus M, Kennell J: *Maternal-infant bonding (The impact of early separation or loss on family development)*. St. Louis, Mosby, 1976.

30. Spitz R, Wolf K: The smiling response: A contribution to the ontogenesis of social relations, *Genetic Psychology Monographs* 34:57–125, 1946.

31. Stern D: Mother and infant at play: The dyadic interaction involving facial, vocal and gaze behavior, in *The effect of the infant on its care giver*. Edited by Lewis M, Rosenblum M. New York: Wiley, pp. 187–215, 1974.

32. Boston Women's Health Collective: *Our bodies, ourselves*, 2nd ed. New York: Simon & Schuster, 1976.

33. Sommer B: The effect of menstruation on cognitive and perceptual motor behavior: A review, *Psychosomatic Medicine* 35 (7):515–534, 1973.

34. Castelnuovo-Tedesco P, Krout B: Psychosomatic aspects of chronic pelvic pain, *Psychiatry in medicine* 1:109–126, 1970.

35. Neugarten B, Kraines R: "Menopausal symptoms" in women of various ages, *Psychosomatic Medicine 27* (3):266–273, 1965.
36. McKinlay S, Jeffreys M: The menopausal syndrome, *British Journal of Preventive and Social Medicine 28* (2):108–115, 1974.
37. Neugarten B: The awareness of middle age, in *Middle age and aging*. Edited by Neugarten B. Chicago, University of Chicago Press, 1968.
38. Katz J: *Past and future of the undergraduate woman*. Paper presented at Radcliffe Precentennial Conference, Cambridge, Mass., April 1978.
39. Veevers J: Voluntary Childlessness: A review of issues and evidence, *Marriage and Family Review 2* (2):1–26, 1979.
40. Campbell A, Converse P, Ridgers W: *The quality of American life*. New York, Russell Sage, 1976.
41. Bernard J: *The future of marriage*. New York, World, 1972.
42. Campbell A: The American way of mating: Marriage si, children only maybe, *Psychology Today*, pp. 37–43, May 1975.
43. Cope P: The women of *Who's Who*: A statistical study, *Journal of Social Forces 7*:212–224, 1928.
44. Kaltreider N, Margolis A: Childless by choice: A clinical study, *American Journal of Psychiatry 134* (2):179–182, 1972.
45. Mazor M: The problem in infertility, in *The woman patient: Medical and psychological interfaces*, Vol. 1, pp. 137–160. Edited by Notman M, Nadelson C. New York: Plenum Press, 1978.
46. Menninger K: Somatic correlations with the unconscious repudiation of femininity in women, *Journal of Nervous and Mental Disease 89*:514–527, 1939.
47. Kipper D, Zigler-Shani Z, Serr D, Incler V: Psychogenic infertility, neuroticism and the feminine role: A methodological inquiry, *Journal of Psychosomatic Research 21* (5):353–358, 1977.
48. Mai F, Rump E: Are infertile men and women neurotic? *American Journal of Psychology 24*:83, 1972.
49. Weisman M, Klerman G: Sex differences and the epidemiology of depression, *Archives of General Psychiatry 34*:98–111, 1977.
50. McDonald R, Gynther M, Christakos A: Relations between maternal anxiety and obstetric complications, *Psychosomatic Medicine 25* (4):357–362, 1963.
51. Meles F, Hamburg D: Psychological effects of hormonal changes in women, *Human sexuality in four perspectives*. Edited by Beach F. Baltimore, Johns Hopkins University Press, 1976.

Chapter 3

Changing Sex Stereotypes: Some Problems for Women and Men

Norman E. Zinberg

> *Interviewer: Mr. Thurber, what do you expect to happen to the relation-*
> *ships between men and women during the next half century?*
> *Thurber: Women will get stronger; men will get weaker; and dogs will*
> *remain about the same.*
> Interview with James Thurber, *The New York Times*, January 1,
> 1950

The new feminism, which originated in 1963 with the publication of Betty Friedan's *The Feminine Mystique*,[1] has had an enormous impact on attitudes as well as behavior. From it has emerged the contention that normative sex roles are culturally relative, that is, that the active and passive functions of personal and socioeconomic life have, within certain biological limits, been divided between the sexes in different ways by different cultures at different times. So swiftly has this feminist contention penetrated the popular imagination that little time has been available to consider the problems that a change in sex roles has created for individual men and women.[2]

My hypothesis in this chapter is that the division between activity and passivity is the chief factor in differentiating between the roles of the sexes. First, I describe the historical development of sex roles in the American culture, culminating in the stereotype of the passive woman, and I relate these stereotyped sex roles to the changing views and theories of sexual activity itself. Next, I show how the roles imposed on the sexes by society are internalized in the superego and ego states of men and women, and I contend that the relationship of the social setting, and its changes, to individual ego states is a neglected area of study in psychoanalytic theory. And finally, I suggest

Norman E. Zinberg, M.D. • Department of Psychiatry, The Cambridge Hospital, Cambridge, Massachusetts.

ways to minimize social and psychological problems if there is to be a transition to egalitarianism between the sexes.

I draw on essentially qualitative data from the study of individual patients, depth interviews from a formal research project,[3] gleanings from historical* and psychoanalytic writings, and long-standing observations of and interviews with members of specific segments of the social setting, such as communes, that can serve as forecasters of potential shifts in attitude within the larger, normative social setting. Obviously, such data vary in depth and do not encompass all segments of the population equally. Although not all the people and situations I have studied were middle class, the data of greatest depth and consistency have come from middle-class patients. Thus, while I believe that many of my theoretical positions have applicability beyond the middle class, I have limited the assumptions about sex roles to that class. At the same time, the data drawn from middle-class patients cannot, of course, be taken as representative of the nonpatient population. Consequently, other material, obtained from nonpatients, has been included, even though my sample of nonpatients is not large enough to correct for middle-class bias. This material is intended not to serve as experimental data but to provide evidence for my hypothesis concerning the problems relating to changes in sex roles. In order to test my hypothesis, procedures far different from those used in my scattered collection of interviews would be required.

THE ACTIVE–PASSIVE DIMENSION

Any discussion of activity–passivity as a dimension should differentiate active or passive behavior from "ego" activity–passivity. For example, a soldier obeying commands thoughtlessly is behaviorally active but ego-passive, while the reverse is true of a scientist actively pondering a knotty problem but scarcely moving a muscle. In the area of sexual stereotyping, the separation of ego activity–passivity from its behavioral counterparts can be very complex. It is clear that any specific feeling or internalized view of self may lead to many different activities in different people, and that at the same time, any specific observable activity may stem from many different feelings or views of the self. But when such things as work and attitudes toward work, or nurturance and its accompanying emotional and cognitive positions, are being considered, people universally have mixed internal feelings.

*My indebtedness to Robinson's *The Modernization of Sex*,[4] Peale's " 'Normal' Sex Roles: An Historical Analysis,"[5] and Thomas's "The Double Standard"[6] for placing my clinical data in an historical and social context goes beyond simply acknowledging them as references.

All of us feel in part active, that is, aggressive, competitive, intrusive, and, in a sense, dominating. But all of us also feel passive, that is, nurturant, tension-regulating, receptive, and, in a sense, submissive. It is how this ambivalence expresses itself in behavior and is proportioned within the individual and in the sex roles developed by the individual and the society that is being considered here.[7]

Thus, few men reject some receptive fantasies about caring and being cared for, and in their working lives, they begin a career by taking orders instead of giving them. While taking orders, they may well be planning and learning how to give them, and while thinking of nurturing a child or a friend, they may well be resisting any show of tenderness. These two passive experiences, as well as many others, are not totally akin. Nevertheless, it is my contention that within the American middle-class social setting, not only are male responses that are generally thought of as passive restricted behaviorally, but the disapproval of the larger culture restricts even the conscious exploration of most passive fantasies. From a very early age, little boys who play with dolls are called "sissies." Few of the building blocks of the conscious identity of young males consist of areas sufficiently unconflicted to permit passive responses, internal and external, to serve the aim of self-esteem and self-confidence. Thus, men are ambivalent about, even suspicious of, *any* passive desires.

Women, on the other hand, partake more freely of both an inner life and external behavior in which activity and passivity are intermixed. Little girls can play active games and also play with dolls if they choose. If "tomboy" behavior does not go too far or persist too late, that label does not carry quite the pejorative meaning of "sissy." Unlike men, whose active goals are clearly directed by society and are expected to exclude other feelings, women must balance both types of feelings and must struggle with the task of finding acceptable limits. However, the questions of where and when activity is permissible and acceptable, and to what degree passive interests may be set aside, cause strong ambivalence. Certainly, the stereotype of wife–mother–homemaker reflects the predominance of a cultural view of the passive-receptive aspects of these functions,[5] although the same stereotype is also "active"; that is, woman's role as homemaker is, in fact, active and administrative but is perceived as passive, in part because of the economic arrangement.

At all stages, however, a variety of active functions is also expected of women. The building blocks of an ego identity permit both active and passive functions to generate the potential for self-esteem and self-confidence. Furthermore, the range of such factors in identity varies to a much greater degree in individual women than among men, for the intricacy of dealing with both functions is affected by differing physical capacities and cultural influences. Thus women are ambivalent not about activity or passivity *per se* but about the *extent* to which each is permissible. As Dr. Grete L. Bibring, the first woman professor of psychiatry in the history of the Harvard Medical School, perceptively stated, "Little boys have more anxieties." (Any passivity arouses fear.) "Little girls have more grievances." (Making decisions about limits makes for tendentiousness.)[8]

THE CULTURAL ACCEPTANCE OF WOMEN AS PASSIVE

The enormous increase in interest in "women" over the last 10 years has produced abundant historical evidence to support the contention that seeing women as stereotypically passive is a relatively recent cultural determination. The growth after World War II of the view that to find "fulfillment," a woman should devote herself to the love, care, and companionship of husband and children at least partly developed from, and was consistently reinforced by, psychological theories stressing the importance of the mother–child relationship and indicating the delicacy of the "mental health" of a child who lacked the overwhelming commitment of its "mother."[2] In the period immediately following World War II, when the woman's role was restricted, such considerations were easily exaggerated, partly in order to give the role of wife–mother–homemaker an aura of importance. Although these pronouncements lacked supporting data, they were seen as authoritative and led to uncertainty and guilt.

Peale's[5] excellent historical analysis of "normal" sex roles in the United States supports my interpretation and offers evidence of previous developments that set the stage for the post–World War II period and for the present rebellion against stereotypes. She showed that the colonial family functioned as an integrated unit: women helped produce supplies, processed the material for garments and fashioned them, prepared for the hard winter, and sometimes even killed Indians. The family unit was not bound by rigid definitions of what was considered woman's work.[9] Families of all classes worked together, which meant that man had a greater role in the direct care of children and other tension-regulating, fostering functions.

Not until the mid-nineteenth century, starting just before but sharply accelerated by the Industrial Revolution, did male–female functions become more sharply separated. Opportunities for commerce and industrial development—the "get-rich-quick" syndrome—led men to leave the family for job opportunities. Cities burgeoned: New York's population increased 10-fold from 1810 to 1860, and· Cin-

cinnati went from 2,500 in 1810 to 160,000 in 1860.[10] Home came to be a place for "board and lodging" for men, and the nuclear family became an increasingly separated and isolated unit. Peale quoted from a book by Graves, popular in 1843, that bemoaned the fact that men were not only totally uninvolved in bringing up their children and saw them only on the Sabbath, but also increasingly recognized no other role for themselves.[11]

Apparently, this acceptance of male–female functional separateness occurred far more swiftly and completely in the United States than in Europe. Traditional social structures and values were already weak in the New World, making further loosening easier.[12] The commercial opportunities that opened for men in the United States with such richness and such promise thrust them directly into the aggressive, competitive marketplace. They were then defined, as people and as men, in terms of their participation in the business world. At the same time, women's assumption of what are now considered the more passive functions of family nurturing, tension regulation, expression of emotion, and guarding of religious and moral values was, in part—perhaps largely—a defensive response. The social change had left a vacuum and had simultaneously removed women from their previous nondifferentiated functions. Peale said, "Women were told explicitly that since they were now useful only as they contributed to the happiness of others, they must consciously cultivate those qualities that made them agreeable."[5]

Despite the extent to which women were asked to assume this stereotyped passive role, they retained more explicitly active functions than did the star-crossed, middle-class group of the late 1940s and 1950s. For one thing, the total separation of functions between men and women left women almost completely autonomous in the home. For another, they served as caretakers of the moral, intellectual, and cultural heritages, and, according to many important European visitors, superior ones at that.[12,13] This period also saw the development of the first feminist movement.[13]

After World War II, however—when the number of household servants decreased, labor-saving devices were introduced, and "culture" was disseminated through the mass media—these active factors were minimized. The return of men from World War II, feeling justified in a search for material security, was not a ripe time psychologically for a feminist movement. Instead, urban middle-class women accepted the passive feminine stereotype of wife–mother and suffered behavioral restrictions possibly unparalleled in history.[14]

The same period saw the rise of social and psychological theories that overwhelmingly reinforced passive, nurturant receptivity as the ideal for women. Freud's responsibility in this area has been much discussed both pro and con.[15,16,17] Certainly, his work provided a basis for extending the biological fact of motherhood and its implications into the development of a separate psychology for women, ascribing to them the passive (even masochistic) functions as innate, and relegating to men the "natural" right to aggression and what Erikson[18] later called "intrusion."

Many psychoanalytic writers, including, interestingly enough, several women—for example, Deutsch,[19] Bonaparte,[20] and Lampl-de Groot[21]—elaborated and fortified this position at the same time that others[22,23] were emphasizing the crucial aspects for childhood development of proper, consistent (full-time), and wholehearted motherhood.

It should be noted that these pressures on women came not from psychoanalysis alone. In 1955, two extremely influential sociologists, Parsons and Bales,[24] stated that the biological reality of females' bearing and nurturing children was the cause of the social-psychological differentiation of sex roles. They described the male role as instrumental-adaptive, which conforms more or less to the activity functions, and the female role as expressive and tension-regulating, which they defined as passive functions. Although unquestionably the role allotted to women in this differentiation has active and adaptive functions, this aspect was minimized by Parsons and Bales, possibly for symmetry, since their discussion of the male role includes few potentially positive aspects of passivity. In a related work Parsons stated that boys, while not understanding the nature of their fathers' work, learn that "it would be shameful to grow up to be like a woman." He made much of the need in American culture for boys to avoid any feminine identification, to develop physical prowess and toughness, and above all to inhibit the expression of any tender (feminine-expressive-passive) emotions.[25]

The list of apostles of the creed of the post–World War II period is very long indeed. In retrospect, the most interesting and important aspect of their allotting the active role so entirely to men and the passive role to women is their unawareness that, in the case of women, they were breaking with the historical tradition of woman's less differentiated functioning. Not only did both sociologists and psychologists overlook much anthropological scholarship that clearly showed that sex roles varied from society to society and within the same society over time,[26] but in a more important way their search for the proper or mentally "healthy" role caused them to overlook the evidence of their own senses. Indeed, during this period of approximately 15 or 20 years, although middle-class, urban women tried very hard to become child-chauffeuring, bread-baking mothers, their search for active, intrusive participation in affairs both within and outside the home never stopped. The incredible growth in the use of women volunteers in hospitals, social agencies, and community affairs is only one indicator of their restlessness. One reason for this oversight, as well as a crucial element in understanding the tenacity of stereotyped sex roles, was the view of sexual activity itself and the failure to recognize that it was undergoing change.

THE DOUBLE STANDARD

Until the advent of "the pill," the physical fact of the potential for pregnancy dominated any consideration of the female role and thus caused it to be sharply differentiated from the male role. Concern about pregnancy influenced and curtailed women's sexual activity for centuries. To quote Dr. Samuel Johnson, "female chastity is of the utmost importance because upon that all the property in the world depends."[27] Bastard children intrude into the husband's inheritance, and it is then a wise father indeed who can know his own child. Hence, the fears of an unwanted pregnancy combined with the fears of the burden placed on society by illegitimacy to reinforce the notion that women *should* be sexually inhibited. Through the Victorian era, this idea developed into the notion that they *were* inhibited and that perhaps it was those who were not sexually passive who were the deviants.

This twisting of the biological differences between the sexes in American culture, which led to the acceptance by both men and women of the necessity for woman's passivity, led more than anything else to an overall obscuring of women's equal identification with active functions. The double standard accepted in sexual relations affected all male–female definitions. And the double standard was indeed accepted, as admirably documented by Keith Thomas.[6] He pointed out that for hundreds of years, it was not only kings and male courtiers who were urged to keep mistresses but the common man as well. As a result, in 1841, the Metropolitan District of London alone had over 4,000 brothels. English law, following its Germanic precursor, made adultery a crime for women but (except for incest) not for men. Well into the latter half of the nineteenth century, a man was entitled to use violence and physical restraint to secure the person and services of his wife, whereas she was able to regain her renegade husband only by means of a court order. All this was justified under English law by the need to protect the property rights of the woman's father or husband.

THE IMPACT OF FREUD'S THINKING

By the end of the nineteenth century, efforts had been made to achieve greater equality under the law for women, and some changes had occurred in social mores. Although it can now be seen that Freud's "anatomy is destiny" strengthened sexual stereotypes in the long run, its initial impact was powerfully liberal.* As has been pointed out repeatedly, Freud was a product of the latter half of the "Victorian century."[30] His patients, too, were products of their time. Most of his early reported cases were women who had severe somatic symptoms that Freud and others labeled as hysterical.[31] Without exception, they were sexually repressed, fearful of sexual thoughts as well as acts. Freud fought that repression; he told them to accept their sexuality and thus be free of their symptoms. Thus, Freud, the prototype of the liberal urge toward sexual freedom, was derided by his peers for his struggle against sexual repression and was attacked as the destroyer of conventional morality. It is ironic to find him berated now as an advocate of sexual repression and middle-class conformity.

At all times, Freud's aim was that women, as well as men, should like and accept themselves, all of themselves, including the repressed and forbidden sexual urges. But he recognized how hard a job this was from both the cultural and the biological perspective. In one of the cases in "Studies on Hysteria,"[31] the woman suffered because, as an employee, her dreams of any intimate relationship to her employer foundered before the rigid Victorian social structures as surely as if she had been biologically of another species. Freud spoke then, as he did often thereafter, of the limiting conditions imposed by society.

Nevertheless, by training, perhaps by inclination, and certainly by cultural background, Freud was inclined to put greater stress on the physiological and biological than on the social factors.[32] His early discovery of the unconscious as a coherent mental structure also immersed him in the most primitive aspects of human personality, those most closely connected to animal forebears and to inborn universal givens. No wonder he believed that at some point a physiological basis must be found for his psychological concepts. But the current criticism of Freud shares with the critics of his own day a lack of appreciation of his view of the human condition. For Freud saw life at all times as a never-ending struggle. The tragic consequences of a rigid class system were clear to him when considering Lucy R.; the tragic

---

*As an analyst I find it difficult to write about Freud objectively; in a sense, I live off the fruits of his genius. In other work, however, I have criticized his errors and limitations[2,28] and I can at least strive for objectivity. The dual problem is to keep Freud in a historical perspective and to separate his philosophical musings from his work derived directly from clinical experience.[29]

consequences of biology seemed equally clear when Dora longed for the freedom allowed the males in the family. But Freud did not limit his awareness of the tragic consequences of biology to females deprived of that precious part so dear to males. The need to fear for that part seemed to him to be a tragic biological consequence that would lead to a different but equivalent conflict stemming from having been born with a biologically irreversible or (until a recent technological advance) determined sex. This pessimistic conviction of Freud's has been distorted, plucked out of its historical context, and reviewed in the light of feminist concerns.

Another problem that preoccupied Freud—and here the charge that he reflected cultural biases is better founded—was masochism.[33] Given a theory that rested on the dualistic instincts of self-preservation and preservation of the race, where did self-destructive, self-hurtful preoccupations originate? After all, trying to understand what pushes people to act against themselves and their own best interests when they are hoping with all their conscious hearts for a good outcome is a vexing puzzle. It is particularly exasperating when the patient participates less well in discussions that are intended to prevent pain than in almost anything else. Clinically, Freud found examples of the need for punishment to expiate guilt or rage at an introjected object. But they never satisfied him, and his philosophic writings turned again and again to this problem. Among women patients, the tendency toward accepting dominance and a lesser, debased view of themselves seemed consistently greater than among men. And here Freud did not look sufficiently to cultural indoctrination for an explanation; instead, he used the idea of masochism (a feminine biological given) as a taking-off point that led to his least tenable idea: a life and death instinct.[34] I think it reasonable to say, given Freud's skeptical curiosity, his willingness to change his mind, and the theme of "Analysis Terminable and Interminable,"[35] that just before his death, he was moving toward a greater interest in cultural relativism and would have reconsidered his position on feminine masochism.

Nevertheless, Freud's belief in the eventual dominance of physiology over psychology and his preoccupation with masochism resulted in his reinforcing the stereotype of the passive female. He never quite saw that his conclusions were the result, rather than the cause, of the double standard.

VIEWS ON SEXUALITY

Writing at the same time and perhaps exerting a greater influence on our thinking about sexuality, though not on general concepts of human psychology, was H. Havelock Ellis.[36] Ellis, called by Robinson[4] the first great sexual modernist, treated sexuality with unyielding tolerance and enthusiasm. Above all, he committed himself against the demonic concept of sexuality held by those scientists before, after, and including Freud who thought of sex as an instinct. Although he was uneasy with Freud's instinct theory and ambivalent about other of Freud's ideas, eventually he found himself in closer agreement with Freud than he wanted to be. One unfortunate area of agreement concerned the natural sexual passivity of women.

Ellis claimed that female sexuality was more passive and more diffuse than male sexuality, that it required more arousal, and that it was essentially receptive. Using examples from animal courtship, he stressed the masculine tendency to dominate and the female delight in submission. This approach permitted him to ground sadistic and masochistic tendencies in normal behavior, which, as Robinson pointed out, was a constant thrust in his work. Nevertheless, while concluding that sadism was only a pathological extension of the normal male sexual psychology and masochism the same for women, his "genuinely empirical treatment" caused him to disagree with Krafft-Ebing's even more forceful statements on the same issue.[37] Krafft-Ebing had insisted that if the usual situation was reversed and a woman was sadistic or a man masochistic, he or she was inevitably a homosexual. When Ellis found no clinical support for this concept, he went further and suggested that even animal courtship showed no clear breakdown of sexual roles along sadistic and masochistic lines.

Ellis, like Freud, however, was preoccupied with motherhood. "It is the mother," he stated, "who is the child's supreme parent." In documenting Ellis's ambivalence toward female sexuality, Robinson pointed out that although Ellis never argued that a woman could be nothing else if she were a mother, the essential tendency of his thought was to confine her to the home. "Women were designed to make children, men to make history," Ellis said.

Had it not been for his enthusiasm for motherhood, there is little doubt that Ellis, whose work foreshadowed that of Masters and Johnson, would not have ended up with so passive a view of woman's sexuality. Robinson stated that Ellis "advocated complete legal, political, and professional equality for women, insisted on their right to authority and independence within the family and defended their claim to equal sexual privileges." Although Ellis's first book on sexual inversion presents six times as many male cases as female, his plea for tolerance toward homosexuality as a simple congenital predisposition and not a form of deviance was aimed equally at both sexes. Moreover, his insistence that masturbation was not linked with physical or mental disturbance—perhaps his greatest demythification—explicitly included women and served to undermine the nineteenth-century belief that women lacked sexuality.

And finally, his essential division of the stages of sexual arousal into tumescence and detumescence was intended to cover both sexes. (His division exactly parallels Masters and Johnson's[38,39] later, more complex, but less experientially sound four-step division of the stages of arousal.) This work[36] came at a time when almost all other studies of human sexuality referred to masculine responses alone. Ellis explained that the vascular congestion (tumescence) and decongestion (detumescence) that accompany orgasm signify the entire process of sexual arousal and release. Thus, he called attention to sexual arousal as a conscious process and a preliminary to every sexual act. After Ellis's work, arousal could be and often was seen as a problem, whereas previously the sole problem had been the control of the powerful, even demonic, sexual urges. By reversing this concern and specifying the necessity for what he called "courtship," Ellis opened the question of responsibility for female frigidity. In fact, by stressing his belief in cultural relativism, he set the stage for later researchers to study the influence of personality and social setting on sexual arousal, just as he did for the study of these same influences on psychoactive drug use.

The paucity of comprehensive and coherent sex research from the turn of the century until after World War II, which may be one indication of social stability, is nevertheless surprising. For this was the time when Henry Ford and his confreres were providing Americans with bedrooms on wheels. Tiny and uncomfortable as it was, the automobile began the great change in sexual mores. Perhaps the most important recognition of the influence of this technological change came in the work of Kinsey.[40,41] Kinsey included what he anachronistically called "petting" as one of the six important sexual outlets. In this instance, as in others, he was accurately reflecting the existing mores; yet he gave the impression that what he was measuring were not highly variable mores much affected by social and technological change but certain almost natural states of sexual being.

Kinsey was a great empiricist as well as a great demystifier of sex. Since orgasms were measurable events, they became his standard regardless of quality or circumstance. He paid little or no attention to such sexual difficulties as transvestism and voyeurism because they seldom led to orgasms. In the same fashion, he reduced heterosexual intercourse to one of a set of acts. His list of outlets included masturbation, nocturnal emission, heterosexual petting, heterosexual intercourse, homosexual relations, and intercourse with animals of other species (the predominant concept of sexual relations was just number four). This entirely empirical approach was not surprising, however,

in a biologist who had previously been chiefly concerned with classi-
fying the gall wasp.[42,43]

Kinsey's extreme pragmatism, making it possible for him to write
that "sex is a normal biological function, acceptable in whatever form
it is manifested," permitted his work to have a remarkably liberalizing
effect on sexual attitudes because it did not appear to be contentious.
Thus, his figures, which showed that 37% of males had had at least
one homosexually induced orgasm, that masturbation was nearly universal, and that social class exerted a powerful influence on sexual
mores, broke through important social pretenses. Kinsey argued re-
lentlessly that we must look at what people actually do sexually, not
what they think they are supposed to do; for only then can we function effectively as sexual beings.

When it came to the differences between men and women, however, Kinsey slipped badly, as Robinson pointed out. Oddly enough,
he knew it, but he did little to reconsider his figures in the light of his
bias. "Comparisons of females and males must be undertaken with
some trepidation and a considerable sense of responsibility," he said,
and he confessed that it would be surprising if he had succeeded in
liberating himself from the prejudices of his upbringing. For example,
he stated that "the average adolescent girl gets along well enough with
a fifth as much sexual activity as the adolescent boy." Aside from his
much criticized exalting of adolescent male sexuality, he neglected his
own data, which showed women to be more sensitive to psychological
influences than men. Although World War I and later developments
had little affected the sexual behavior of men but had had a substantial
impact on female sexual behavior, Kinsey still accepted the proposition that the differences between male and female behavior were biologically determined. As is revealed by a close reading of *Sexual Behavior in the Human Female*,[41] he treated his own findings about female
sexuality, including the statistical, with little rigor.

And the biological differentiation to which Kinsey clung found
women's sexuality inherently passive and thus less sensitive to psychological stimuli than men's. The male, in both animals and humans,
according to Kinsey, initiated the sexual activity, proving that the male
was more inclined to experience sexual response before making actual
physical contact. He insisted on this position despite the finding that
some women could achieve orgasm by fantasy alone, while none of
his more than 9,000 male subjects reported a similar achievement. By
deciding that sex for women was more a physical than an emotional
reality, Kinsey, as Robinson pointed out, ironically reversed the stereotyped belief that chained women sexually because of their hyper-

emotionality. But this reversal was necessary for Kinsey because it explained men's higher rates of sexual outlet. He simply could not concede that pressures from the social setting shaped female psychology. Along with Ellis, he argued that men's greater interest in sexual variety developed directly from their more active capacities, a finding not to be refuted for 20 years. As a result of this conclusion, Kinsey stated explicitly that the double standard, which allotted the passive, accepting role to women, was firmly grounded in natural psychological differences between the two sexes.

Toward the end of his life, Kinsey began to think in terms of sexual experimentation, but he believed that as yet this was culturally unacceptable. That his belief was correct can be deduced from the furor caused when Masters and Johnson's pioneering efforts were published in 1966.[38] By that time, however, the emotional climate surrounding sex had become more liberal (partly as the result of Kinsey's work), and Masters and Johnson could survive the uproar. Their work reflected both a growing cultural awareness that little was known about either the physiology or the psychology of sex and a disenchantment with the Victorian moral hangover that accepted such ignorance. It helped to prepare the United States for the far-reaching reassessment of male–female sex roles.

Robinson took Masters and Johnson to task for their prose. He contended that their turgid, opaque, and sloppy writing masks the imprecision of their thinking and veils the conservative ideology that appears in their work, even when they are considering their experimental material. In this I concur, as I do with his contention that this couple, by combining their shocking empirical experimentation with a romantic preoccupation with monogamy,[44] could gain respectability. A clearer, more precise scientist would probably have been dismissed as heartless. Nevertheless, in a rare disagreement with Robinson, I think that at the time that Masters and Johnson's work first appeared, their very unintelligibility convinced the general public of their scientific integrity, thus providing another case of the acceptance of stereotyping. Furthermore, it veiled the fact that they were naive psychological clinicians who suffered from what their primary antagonist, Freud, called excessive therapeutic ambition.

Nevertheless, their work illuminated sexual functioning (particularly that of the human female), corrected the misconceptions of centuries, and fueled the feminist movement. Their experimental work and their later therapeutic posture insisted on the female potential for sexual activity. It was the perfect antidote to Kinsey's view of biologically passive femininity. Masters and Johnson showed that the female, in many periods of the life cycle, has a greater actual sexual capacity than the male and that the only sexual inhibitions against activity are social. Under laboratory conditions and when it was explicitly indicated to be acceptable, their female subjects could and would be directly aggressive and initiatory both in behavior and in fantasy.

In particular, Masters and Johnson's work on masturbation—it could more properly be called a celebration of masturbation—was principally confined to women, in sharp contrast to Kinsey's work. Not only did they claim that masturbation during menstruation relieves menstrual pain, but also they ambiguously recommend masturbation for postmenopausal women because those older women who do not masturbate regularly "often have difficulty in accommodating the penis during their rare exposures to coition." This comment calls attention not to the older women's reduced desire but—and remember that Masters and Johnson approach sex almost exclusively from the set of monogamy—to older men's reduced performance. In fairness, I should add that their emancipation of female sexuality, great as that achievement is, may be secondary in the long run to their enfranchisement of sex for both men and women in the later decades of life.

Their suggestion that masturbation may actually be superior to intercourse may seem to conflict with their glorification of marital monogamy, but they square that contradiction in their sexual therapy. There they use essentially masturbatory techniques as training for successful coition, and there is a definite implication that these techniques may continue to be necessary or important. Thus, even in the process of achieving heterosexual satisfaction, some aspects of masturbation remain supreme. It would be more exact to point out that in their therapy, it is principally the female who is the sexually active "therapist." She both directs the man in showing him how to satisfy her and is in charge of manipulating him. This accentuation is so pronounced that Robinson facetiously suggested that Masters and Johnson's books be retitled *Female Sexual Response* and *Male Sexual Inadequacy*.

However it is stated, whether in a description of their experiments or of their therapy, Masters and Johnson's emphasis on the satisfaction of masturbation for the female clearly tends to liberate women from their sexual dependence on men. A woman can be both sexually active and passive, whether in relation to herself or in relation to others. A man, however—and his situation has never been more sharply defined than in their writings—is expected to be active in successful sexual relationships even though he may often fail in the attempt. Woman's failure, then, is a male responsibility, and she must teach him how to allow her to succeed. The implication is that once she is aware of her prowess and accepts it, she will not often fail; and thus she can succeed sexually on both the active and the passive level. Masters and Johnson quarreled overtly with the Freudian concept of clitoral and vaginal orgasms, and they indicated many ways in which women can achieve satisfaction. Not so for the man. His only passive role is as the tutee of the woman, based usually on his sexual inadequacy—a situation that he is supposed to overcome and not one easily accepted as a source of self-esteem and self-confidence.

Thus, woman's capacity for both activity and passivity has finally been recognized, both in the work place and, as a result of Masters and Johnson's findings, in the bedroom. In the work place, that dual capacity has long been acknowledged; in fact, the increased and excessive denial of woman's active functioning in the period following World War II was an historical accident brought about by the conditions created by the war and reinforced by a new and powerful psychological approach. Although it was a short-lived period, it may well have fueled the female bitterness and impatience so important in the current feminist movement. In the bedroom, on the other hand, the repression of woman's active side has a longer, deeper history. Here, too, however, the modernization of ideas about sex, partly as a result of the technology that made Masters and Johnson's experiments possible and partly through the development of the pill, has shown the foolishness of seeing women as exclusively passive.

The Activity–Passivity Conflict

To a certain extent, the long-held social view of the passive woman has affected each woman's view of herself—of her identity. But each woman has also had experiential knowledge of her capacity for action, and in many of life's activities, she has found ways to gain esteem and confidence through that part of her nature. Even those women who found, and unfortunately still find, themselves frigid and sexophobic because of the conflict between their sexual potential and their view of what is sexually proper, by the very nature of that conflict have an awareness of their active bent. Thus, the woman's conflict about activity has had to do less with the question of whether to accept it as an intrinsic, satisfying, esteemed part of herself than with a concern about where and when her active bent was reasonable and proper. In psychoanalytic terms, this is more a conflict within the superego or between the superego and the ego than a conflict within the ego. Saying this does not, of course, minimize the dehabilitating nature of such a conflict. Any one of us who has experienced the painful guilt (and who has not?) that comes from violating a lifelong commandment or not living up to a treasured archetype knows the proportion of such guilt and the range of behavior and labyrinthine inner mechanisms devised to avoid it. The superego, however, is directly dependent on social cues for nurturance; it is a curious mixture of archaic rigidity and all-too-convenient flexibility. Even late in life, changes in the social environment can rather quickly bring about changes in our internal view of what is permissible. Hence, if the chief conflict about activity for women is a superego conflict, the social acceptance of the feminist movement's ideals should be rather readily incorporated into the psychology of individual women.

Not so for men. My reading of recent history, for both the work place and the bedroom, indicates that the little boy who is made to feel ashamed of his interest in dolls finds little in later life to contradict that judgment. At least since the Industrial Revolution, any esteem accruing to him, from both the inside and the outside, has resulted from his capacity to actively master aspects of his social environment. He has fully accepted the expectation that he be the breadwinner: even to chance the more passively labeled possibilities of achieving that aim has carried the risk of ridicule. Nichols and May's record "My Son the Nurse"[45] achieved hilarity by satirizing a man's desire for success in a "woman's profession." And certainly, there was no surcease for him in bed. He was expected to perform actively, and although the word *perform* has recently become a pejorative, those psychiatrists who have seen an increasing number of male patients complaining of impotence[46] recognize how vital to these individuals is their ability to function in bed at all times. The inhibition of men's passive interests does not relate so much to where or when passive interests may be expressed as to whether they may be expressed at all. Where in American society, in fact, can men (except for the relatively few social workers, dynamic psychiatrists, and possibly some teachers) achieve satisfaction, gain esteem, and increase self-confidence through passive interests? Passive wishes are not just forbidden as wrong; they are specifically not accepted by the ego as useful aspects of the male's sense of himself. Thus, dealing with them involves an ego conflict, not, as with women, a predominantly superego conflict.

The rate of change involved in ego development, unlike that in superego development, is extremely slow, requiring perhaps several generations. It seems, therefore, that the psychologies of men and women are now changing at vastly different rates. If this difference is not understood and allowed for, the danger of a major escalation of the war between men and women is very great. I have already indicated the crucial role played by the social setting in determining these changes in both the ego and the superego. Now I will spell out the theoretical basis for this statement, which will show that the relationship between the social setting and individual ego states has been a neglected area of study in psychoanalytic theory.

RELATION TO PSYCHOANALYTIC THEORY

Generally speaking, Freud's great discovery of the unconscious continues to dominate psychoanalytic theory. Freud's interest gradually moved from a concern with primitive unconscious forces (the timeless, primordial id) to a concern with how these forces are tamed and used in everyday life (the mediating, balancing ego). Most psychoanalytic theorists have followed this pattern, placing particular emphasis on early development. Certainly, in the studies of the early years, the relationships with significant others have received consistent and careful attention. It is assumed, however, that these early relationships are effectively internalized, even though often ambivalently, and thus, that they act as precursors of an organized identity. Because these early internalized relationships are critical factors in the emergence of the ego as relatively autonomous from the id, throughout life they remain very closely connected to and influenced by the primitive, undifferentiated impulses of the id. Hence, in effect, the more recent object-relationship approaches to psychoanalytic theory, which take the external environment into account as a powerful influence, do so from a vantage point similar in perspective to the original stance of psychoanalytic theory.[47,48,49,50,51]

By stressing so heavily the external relationships that are internalized in childhood, which are deeply unconscious and timelessly fixed, psychoanalytic theory is continuing to focus on the way in which primitive forces—albeit now not so directly biological—are mediated by the ego. Yet, not until 1937 did Freud himself explicitly indicate that significant external events might become crucial to the stability of the ego and that, indeed, innumerable latent conflicts might become manifest throughout life under certain social circumstances.[35] Erikson greatly enlarged this theme,[18] but he, too, was bound by a preoccupation with early development. Although he was fully aware of the relationship between essential personality configurations and later life interactions with the external world, his original schema in *Childhood and Society*, which formed the basis of all his later work, was rooted in the libido theory. Rapaport[52] lamented the lack, in psychoanalytic theory, of a systematic consideration of the influence of the social setting on the continuing development and maintenance of relative ego autonomy. And his work,[7] along with that of others,[28,53,54,55] laid the theoretical groundwork for a consideration of these influences.

Rapaport agreed that

> To understand how the ego, whose functions determine and delineate a sense of self, remains relatively autonomous and copes with the demands of the external environment and of the basic, inborn forces Freud termed "instinctual drives" requires consideration of both [the external environment and the inborn forces] and their interactions.[52]

The autonomy Rapaport postulated is always relative, and the inside drives and the outside environment carefully balance each other.

Rapaport told the story of the man who did not march in step to an enthralling military band because he was pondering, and he pointed out how falling in love saved Orwell's protagonist of *1984*,[56] at least temporarily, from the press of that overwhelming environment. The drives thus prevent man from becoming a stimulus–response slave.

On the other side, the continuous, varied input from the external environment—which Rapaport saw as the stimulus nutriment necessary to sustain the ego—mediates and moderates the primitive drives. Here, Rapaport used the story of Moses and the great king who had been told by his seers and phrenologist that Moses was cruel, vain, and greedy. On finding Moses gentle, wise, and compassionate, the king planned to put his wise men to death. Moses demurred, saying, "They saw truly what I am. What they could not see was what I have made of it."

The input from external reality not only sustains primary ego functions, such as motor capacity, thinking, memory, perceptual and discharge thresholds, and the capacity for logical communication, but also nurtures those secondary ego apparatuses, such as competence, cognitive organization, values, ideals, and a mature conscience. Thus, the individual's capacity to function adaptively in a given cultural setting rests on an interdependence between primitive drives and external environment. They each guarantee his or her ego's relative autonomy from the other. And each, therefore, can be disrupted by disrupting the other.

When the biological process of puberty raises drive to peak tension, adolescents try

> to combat their tendency to subjectivity, seclusiveness, and rebellion by the external, reality-related converse of these—intellectualization, distance from primary objects, and efforts at total companionship. But it is an unequal and often painful struggle. . . . When, as in a concentration camp, external conditions maximize the individual's sense of danger and arouse fears and neediness, the drives no longer act as guarantors of autonomy from the environment, but prompt surrender.

Throughout his discussion Rapaport insists that the superego in particular is dependent on consistent stimulus nutriment. The convention, or American Legionnaire, syndrome—when moderate, respectable men and women remove themselves from their usual routines and social relationships and behave in an impulsive and uncontrolled manner—makes it clear how heavily the strictures of conscience depend on social structure.[28]

In American culture, men receive a highly specific input of stimulus nutriment from the environment, urging them to behave actively and to internalize this active view of themselves. If they deviate from that position, the social input available to them is a generally negative view of themselves. The extent to which the culture has both demanded and rewarded an active posture in males has made somewhat possible the ego's relative autonomy from the id. A concerted effort has been made to dampen passive impulses by neither stimulating nor rewarding them. Obviously, they exist, but in the past, psychoanalysts' efforts to pay attention to the male envy of women's capacity for receptivity and nurturance have paled before the clear evidence that seeking such gratifications would interfere with the ego's relative autonomy from the external environment. Thus, men have become excessively sensitive to external cues and to the relationships that supply these cues.

One price of this increased dependence on the environment has been some impairment of the male ego's relative autonomy from the id. Men's efforts to maintain coherent object relations that permit some balance between activity and passivity are uneasy and sometimes threatening. They agonize constantly about their ability to maintain such relationships and, with some pain, they cling to the stereotyped views of themselves.

CLINICAL ILLUSTRATIONS: TWO MEN

Mr. S

Mr. S, a man in his 40s who had pursued an active, successful career, found himself undone by the feelings stirred up when his wife left him. On careful examination, he discovered that he had constructed his life so that active involvements with male friends predominated. Playing cards, golfing, making deals, serving on boards, and playing around with other women were all sources of gratification and were all done in male company. In each instance, his view of himself and others' views of him as an aggressive but likable man of the world went unchallenged. Aside from his wife, his consistent relationships with women were either with secretaries, housekeepers, or courtesans. He even conducted social repartee in a joking, flirting, edged manner. None of these carefully controlled, distant interactions interfered with his active view of himself, although he was conscious of his discomfort with women. Even with his children, Mr. S maintained a similar stance. He was aware of his discomfort, but the care that went into controlling relationships in order to avoid conflict with his conscious view of himself was itself unconscious.

His relationship with his wife, on the other hand, was consciously ambivalent. He respected her capacity for activity but devoted enormous energy to trying to force her to keep it within a sphere acceptable to him. Her single, brief affair shortly after their marriage had precipitated his one previous period of overwhelming anxiety. His discovery of it and her guilt gave him the right to a hostile dominance, a weapon to keep her in her place. Mr. S used it constantly, subtly, and effectively for 20 years. Her decision to use her active talents more directly outside the home, however, forced him into unusual and excessive uses of this weapon, destroying its effectiveness. His subsequent rages led her eventually to leave him. Suddenly he was flooded with long-repressed, dependent longings and at the same time a dim awareness of the extent to which his marriage had served him as a platform from which to relate to other men. Now, frightened not only by the loss of the one figure on whom he had allowed himself to become emotionally dependent (a dependence masked as hostility), but also by the possibility that these same passive longings could be transferred to men, Mr. S became painfully and overtly anxious.

Mr. B

Young Mr. B, a 20-year-old, handsome college junior from a traditional middle-class background, proud of his athletic accomplishments, reported that as a freshman he had had his first sexual experience with a girl he had come to know fairly well in class. When he decided to pursue her and ask for a date, he was pleased by his own initiative. They went to bed on their first date after an evening that he had experienced as close, intimate, and moving. He was shocked in the morning when his assumption of a continuing relationship was shattered by her easy response, "How nice, but I'll be busy for the next few weeks because my boyfriend is returning." During the next two years, two or three further experiences with young women who saw their sexuality as active, distant, and reminiscent of the male "scoring" stereotype of the 1950s revealed to him the depth of his conviction that the male should be the active seeker after romance. His increasing anxiety on dates, which made him feel insecure and unsure as to how to behave, eventually resulted in impotence, to his excruciating embarrassment. His girlfriends' condescension and sympathy for his plight only compounded his unhappiness.

Mr. B became aware that his basic view of himself as successful harked back to his athletic, social, and intellectual prowess in secondary school and earlier. Without undue arrogance, he had believed himself to be something of a leader of men and women. Now, to feel himself not only a follower of these women—that position he could have tolerated—but the passive recipient of women's favors stirred up the unacceptable wish to play just such a passive role. Though not quite conscious, such thoughts had come close enough to the surface to cause him painful anxiety.

On this count, Mr. B's problem comes close to the modern dilemma being explored in this chapter. As an intelligent young man well versed in psychological theory, he could not escape a nagging concern about his selection of girlfriends. Did he choose exceedingly aggressive women, and did such choices say something about his secret wishes for passivity?

He also discovered that his conscious espousal of male–female egalitarianism had been only a general acceptance of the principle; he had never believed it applied to him personally. Hence, when he became anxious with the women he usually selected to take out, trying to choose those who he thought would not challenge him, or when he retreated to a more monastic existence by studying or playing ball with his buddies, the doubts about his masculinity that began to plague him could not be stilled.

DISCUSSION OF THE MALE CLINICAL ILLUSTRATIONS. The clinical cases of Mr. S and Mr. B fit Rapaport's formulation of a regressive state. As Rapaport put it,

> A regressive state should develop when the ego is unable to maintain its relative autonomy from the id or the external environment. In such a state the barriers differentiating ego and id processes become fluid. Images, ideas, and fantasies based on primary process thinking rise to consciousness, and there develops a reliance on more and more primitive defenses. The sense of voluntariness and of having inner control of one's actions in relation to oneself and to the external environment disappears.[7]

In both Mr. S and Mr. B, the reliance on the external environment to help the ego minimize the pressure from unacceptable unconscious wishes proved excessive because of attitude changes in the social setting or the external environment. These attitude changes resulted in different and less satisfactory stimulus nutriment available to the ego, thus impairing the ego's autonomy from the id. In turn, the minimized autonomy from the id forced each individual to minimize his interactions with the external environment for fear that such interactions would further reduce the barriers between ego and id; that is, they would impair ego autonomy from the external environment. Both men suffered constantly from doubts about their ability to maintain coherent relationships with significant figures in their external environment, causing them to retreat and cling to stereotyped views of themselves. For example, they reduced their interactions with both men and women to situations they could see as nonthreatening. For Mr. S, this meant only business contacts and the most superficial social contacts; for Mr. B, it meant men in his dorm with whom he could play ball or go to the movies, but not his roommates and close friends. Both men's efforts to continue relationships that permitted their stereotypes of themselves to remain intact made them more dependent on external cues that maximized the ego's autonomy from the id. While this maximization afforded them some short-term relief from anxiety, it was at the cost of minimizing the conscious input and trust in the affective and ideational signals that usually regulate judgment and decision, that is, at the cost of impairing the ego's autonomy from the environment. Both men felt isolated from many of their own useful emotions and from certain changing views of the external world that would permit an acceptable, revised sense of self to emerge or a capacity to perceive and integrate what they saw as a changed "objective" reality. Filled with doubts, they further restricted relationships to those aspects of the external environment less likely to present the changed "reality."

Unfortunately, the study of lives precludes controlled experimentation: there is no way to prove that changes in the social setting caused latent conflicts in Mr. S and Mr. B to become manifest or that this would not have happened in a different social setting. The lack of experimental evidence, however, does not mean that we must abandon our good sense and ignore an accumulation of clinical data. My explanation may not be the correct one or the only one, but the data are such that continued study of the influences of the social setting on personality development, particularly the study of sex roles, is essential.

Clinical Illustrations: Two Women

The clinical examples of Ms. Y and Ms. D indicate that women are caught up in the same historical currents as men.

Ms. Y

Ms. Y was an attractive, 42-year-old, married mother of four, whose youngest had gone away to boarding school at 17. When her children were at home, Ms. Y had run an efficient household, been in charge of volunteer fund-raising at a local hospital, and managed to acquire an M.A. degree on a part-time basis. Just after her youngest daughter had gone to boarding school, Ms. Y found her volunteer activities paling and decided that she wanted a real job. The idea of getting paid for what she did became a matter of great importance in spite of the fact that, as her husband pointed out to her, they did not need the money. She also found in herself increasing wishes for such direct rewards for her accomplishments as recognition and status.

Her initial efforts at job-seeking were desultory. Nevertheless, a man she had met through her hospital activities offered her a full-time fund-raising job. Mr. Y, who had supported his wife's ambitions to this point, balked—even panicked—at the idea of the full-time job. He had looked forward to the children's being out of the house so that he and Ms. Y could travel more on vacations and to her accompanying him on business trips. Her idea of a full-time job interfered with his longings for a more leisurely life. They talked and talked, and she began the job. Eventually, he came around, but she felt shaken and guilty, with a sense that she must bring their lives as close to his dream as possible.

Ms. Y found the work itself fulfilling and fascinating. Again and again, she was struck by the difference between a paid and a volunteer job in terms of responsibility and gratification. Nevertheless, several problems emerged. Her old friends clearly resented her working: she was unavailable for lunch, tennis, advice, and company, and their resentment (and what she later suspected to be jealousy) upset her. In addition, she missed the old, easy interactions. These difficulties were compounded by the toughness and brittleness of many of her professional colleagues. She began to be concerned that she was becoming like them: "Without women's lib I would never have been able to stand up to Jim (her husband), but I thought I could work in a man's world without having to stop being a woman. Some of the tough broads I meet every day look and act like lesbians even if they're not. Is that what is going to happen to me?"

Unfortunately, standing up to Jim once had not been a permanent solution. Every month brought a new request, always reasonably stated, for her to join him somewhere, or a new complaint about the decline of their social life because of her work. Each stirred up a fresh conflict and increased anxiety, so that she found herself more and more uneasy when going to work.

In thinking through what made these life changes so painful, Ms. Y discovered how fearful she was that she could not be freely active in what she regarded as a directly competitive situation without becoming destructive. Unconsciously, she was afraid that by not supporting her husband's wishes, she would cause him to have a heart attack. There was room for only one active member in the family, and if it were she, he would be unmanned or destroyed. The idea that a balance could exist between work life and social life surprised her. Just as she had tried to be a 100% wife-mother, now she was trying to be a 100% androgynous worker. Although clearly the work situation had stirred up wishes to be a complete, active woman, much of her discomfort at work came from the problem of achieving a balance. Work not only had raised fears that she would become too masculine but had also revived heterosexual fantasies about men she met and competitive fantasies about other women. Her fears of masculinity were used in part to protect her from such fantasies, which she dreaded would lead to overt acts, both of which she felt to be inappropriate.

In each instance, Ms. Y ran into her tendency to think of things in 100%-or-zero, either–or terms of right and wrong. To a much greater extent than she had imagined, but consonant with the structure of her family of origin, she had constructed her life so as to avoid having to balance activity and passivity in ways that would challenge her traditional view of being a "good" woman. Any activity that went beyond the limit could then never be controlled, and she would have to completely abandon her passive interests and gratification. If she were not entirely good, she would inevitably be entirely bad.

Ms. D

Ms. D, a quiet, contained, efficient young woman who had recently graduated from an excellent college, was torn between marriage and a career. She had been living for two years with a young man who now wished to marry her because he had to leave the area for an academic appointment. This appointment occurred at the same time that a local law school accepted her, after having rejected her the previous year. She was so torn by the need to make a decision that she lost any interest in sex and became increasingly withdrawn from her boyfriend.

Ms. D wanted desperately to have both law school and marriage. Her parents, on the other hand, thought she was addled not to get married and go to a graduate school out west. They did not understand either her intense desire to enter this particular law school or how slim her chances

were to get into another school just as good. Her parents' and her boyfriend's lack of interest in the local law school increased her anxiety because she secretly cared a great deal about this symbol of her excellence.

Just as Ms. Y had believed in all or nothing, Ms. D feared that if she
postponed marriage for even a year, she would never marry. Her desire for
status would leave no room for receptivity or sharing, and her withdrawing from her boyfriend made this a self-fulfilling prophecy. In her eyes,
once her career interests were exposed, no man would come near her, and
women would either fear her or worship her—the latter as frightening as
the former. No balance seemed possible between total activity, which
seemed like aggressive destructiveness, and total passivity, which meant
being reduced to an appendage to a man. If she did not remain a thoroughly good girl and do as her parents and boyfriend wished, which would
leave her stagnant, the active or monster part of her would take over completely and she would not be able to save herself from badness.

DISCUSSION OF FEMALE CLINICAL ILLUSTRATIONS. With the women, the
painful conflict came from their views of themselves as bad (a superego conflict), while the men experienced their greatest pain from their
shaken capacity to use the defenses that maintained their usual sense
of themselves (an ego conflict). Both of the women exhibited ego conflicts intrinsic to their views about unconscious impulses. Seeing
aggression as destruction and passivity as a form of soul death are not
exclusively superego conflicts.

Similarly, there is no doubt that Messrs. S and B believed in-
tensely that their passive longings were morally wrong and bad. But
in the cases of Ms. Y and Ms. D, these conflicts within the ego and
between the ego and the id appeared prominently as a result of the
conflict between ego and superego. The sources of stimulus nutriment
available to them were varied, as they were not for Messrs. S and B.
Getting into a prestigious law school and succeeding at a different job
represented husky chunks of social support. But this support then precipitated a conflict between basic areas of relatedness to the external
environment. It was not so much that the egos of the two women
minimized the relative ego autonomy from the external environment
as that they had to achieve a new balance between elements within
the external environment. Both women developed manifest conflicts
focusing on the men in their lives. These projections on men stood for
both women's own passive interests and satisfactions, but it is also
clear that the men offered themselves as excellent reciprocals for such
projections. While primitive destructive fantasies emerged that represented a minimization of the ego's relative autonomy from the id, there
was no extreme withdrawal from the external environment that would
maximize the ego's relative autonomy from the id.

Thus, no further diminution of the relative autonomy from the id
followed, which would have reduced the barriers between ego and id.

Generally speaking, there was no slipping to the more primitive defenses that characterized Messrs. S and B's need to minimize their relatedness to significant others. Rather than slipping into a stereotype, the women were struggling with a social stereotype that had been internalized, in large measure by their superegos. Each one believed it wrong to break out of the stereotype, and the destructive fantasy toward a man that followed was in part a wish but also in part a further effort of the superego in its alliance with the id to push her back to the proper and idealized path of the exclusive wife–mother. Each was not so much dependent on external cues as she was having trouble deciding which cues remained valid. At no point did she surrender contact with affective and ideational signals, although the conflict aroused by conflicting signals caused great pain. Thus, each ego maintained relative contact with, as well as relative autonomy from, the id. Ms. D's sexual inhibition, for example, disappeared as soon as her boyfriend told her that he was willing to postpone marriage for a year to see how she liked law school. This decision meant to her that she was about to perceive and integrate "objective" reality.

GENERAL PSYCHOANALYTIC OBSERVATIONS

In psychoanalytic writing, it is very difficult to describe the parts of the mental apparatus—superego, ego, and id—without making them sound like concrete wheels, pistons, or speedometers, or worse, without falling into the anthropomorphism and making the divisions of the mental apparatus sound like the person. No one has ever seen or mapped an ego. Also, trying to spell out the factors influencing relative ego autonomy begins to sound mechanistic. At times, these difficulties appear great enough to warrant abandoning psychoanalytic theory and relying on an entirely descriptive approach without any psychoanalytic terms. I finally decided against the second approach. Psychoanalytic theory remains the most comprehensive theory of psychological functioning ever devised. Many of its concepts have been so accepted and internalized by individuals and members of the various academic disciplines that they no longer realize the origin of many notions in general use. The idea that there are often mixed motives in conflict, some of which are not consciously available, or the notion that there are sequences and hierarchies in mental functioning and development, just as there are in physiological functioning and development, is hardly recognized as psychoanalytic. Hence, working within an established framework, even one that lacks a systematic integration of the influence of the changing social setting, means that the issues raised will be discussed within a body of knowledge and not simply treated idiosyncratically. Therefore, I believe, if the issues raised in this chapter prove to have merit, they are more likely to work their way into general awareness. And in my opinion the most vital need in solving the problem of sex stereotyping is for people—both men and women—to be aware that the changing social setting directly affects their personality development, both as children and as adults. If this proposition is accepted, then people will automatically question how this effect occurs and, at each historical moment, what the precipitating issues are.

INFLUENCE OF THE SOCIAL SETTING

Trying to understand the determinants of changing sex stereotypes in order to minimize the war between the sexes is not the only situation that requires focusing on the individual's response to a shifting social environment. In recent years, there have been other activities that, while not as basic to all human functioning as the relationships between the sexes, have stirred up great public anxiety, which anxiety became a crucial aspect of the developing situation. I have shown elsewhere that to understand the effect of psychoactive drugs as well as a person's motive for trying them, one must take three factors into account: the psychopharmacology of the drug itself; the set of the person, including her or his personality configuration; and the physical and social environment in which the use takes place.[57] Recent social events, such as the drug revolution of the mid-1960s and the use of heroin in Vietnam, made it necessary to assess the predominance of the first two variables and the impact of the third. For in these instances, at least, it was the setting that seemed of overriding importance. At the same time, these same critical social events pressured psychiatrists into a reexamination of the conscious mind. Once it became clear that it was not necessarily the deep, unconscious, primitive motives that caused people to try certain psychoactive drugs, it was necessary to reassess the users' conscious experiences with these drugs. In effect, people's conscious experiences affected unconscious conflicts and modified them, rather than the reverse. That is, as people understood better their conscious experiences with drugs, drug use aroused less unconscious fear of ego dissolution and made the possibility of consciousness change a reasonable and less threatening notion.

It is possible that a similar process will occur in relation to sex stereotyping. Until recently, by overlooking the role of the social setting in determining many aspects of sex-related functioning, it was possible to see culturally determined aspects of sexuality as natural, that is, biologically determined or determined so early in life and so thoroughly internalized as to be fixed for life. Obviously, much of sexual identity does rest on biological differences. Equally obviously, the imprinting of cultural standards begins with that first pink or blue bow, and the reiteration of these standards during the early, impressionable years becomes an intrinsic part of each of our identities as men and women. But the traditional view seems to stop there and not to recognize the potential impact of changes in the social setting on mores, attitudes, and eventually on personality. The influence of Freud alone cannot explain that shortsightedness.

Pragmatist Kinsey, for example, insisted on downgrading any historical influence on sexual behavior. In his first volume on men, he went to considerable lengths to show that there had been little change in American sexual habits after World War I. Even when the evidence in his second volume on women indicated specifically that sexual mores were fluid, he minimized the historical pattern he had discovered because it conflicted with his contention that women were sexually less conditionable and more passive than men. This belief, for him as for much of our society, was an article of faith.

The resistance to seeing the social setting as a malleable, intrinsic factor in social change can be explained by our devotion to the status quo. Change is hard; all too often the devil we do not know is more frightening than the one we know. That status quo had something for us: it solved a problem, it presented a way, it served a need. Not only is it hard to recognize and give up solutions that no longer work; it is also hard to acknowledge the extent of our clinging to the status quo against our expressed wishes, as can be seen in the four preceding clinical examples. We wish to be able to change readily and rationally. When we find that painful, we can all too easily conclude that such change is unnecessary or impossible.

However, if we are to avoid an intensified war between the sexes, we must be fully aware of mutual problems. Women have suffered from centuries of unwillingness on the part of a man's world to permit them to express their active side, and this problem continues. Men are beginning to suffer from unwillingness on the part of both men and women to permit men to find acceptable ways to express their passivity. Awareness of problems does not *per se* change attitudes, but it is a necessary first step.

There is the fear that once we begin to chart the influence of the social setting, the demand for social engineering will be irresistible. While the emphasis here is on noting the influence of social change, it is obviously a short step to prescribing such changes. I wish to suggest that society make an effort to build more niches for men to find gratifying work and self-esteem in passive pursuits. I intend this to be a general recommendation, not an exact prescription, such as Skinner's suggestions on how to train or mold individuals in a certain predetermined way.[58] Nevertheless, the push for ever more specific social engineering must be guarded against, just as changing the status quo must be based on a recognition of its prior usefulness.

When there is an awareness that the rate of change for men toward sexual egalitarianism may be markedly slower than for women, a subtle question of tolerance and rationality arises. Obviously, this notion could be misused to protect continued male chauvinism and to slow the rate of change generally. The problem will be to find a pace for society and for individuals that allows change without destruction. To differentiate men who want to put and keep women down from those who are struggling to keep a sense of self together in order to change will be a hard task but not an impossible one.

It is obvious as well that despite momentary losses or gains for, say, the Equal Rights Amendment, the thrust of history is toward egalitarian sex roles. Psychologically, this thrust should benefit men as much as women. The powerful repression of passive interests in men has been extremely costly. Many burn out as a result of their relentless activity. Many more find less and less satisfaction in what they do and struggle with their sense of missing the possibility of greater openness and relaxation. Although physiologically there is no male menopause, it is as valid a clinical syndrome as are the increased nervousness and increased sexual difficulties of adolescent males. Attention must be paid to what is happening to the men. My wish is not for a change of pace in this shift toward sexual egalitarianism but rather that men be allowed to participate in it.

Some measures have been taken already. Enlightened corporations and individuals have begun to recognize the value of midlife career shifts. Almost invariably, these shifts permit men to move from more active, competitive situations to human service. These second careers stress tension regulation and receptivity to social difficulty. Very often, the new jobs are those that used to be considered women's: teaching, nursing, or social services. But such job changes in middle life—which could almost be considered occupational therapy for men— are only a small beginning. Younger men starting out will need full career incentives if they are to undertake new situations that will permit self-esteem and confidence to be derived from passive situations. Obviously, they cannot have children, but they can, for example, run nursery schools or be homemakers, just as women can move into engineering and truck-driving if they wish. For that to happen, the passively oriented occupations must be upgraded financially and socially for both men and women.

As far as direct sexual activity goes, the changes are enormous. Just as it is documented that psychiatrists see more sexually anxious young men,[46] I believe that we are also seeing fewer sexually anxious young women. Some women feel that they are being forced to accept a standard of considerable sexual activity before they are psychologically ready, but the paucity of complaints about frigidity is marked. Despite Kinsey, counting the increased number of female orgasms probably does say something about changing sexual attitudes, but other changes in mores are also leading to freer behavior. Women clearly feel easier about initiating sexual activity, particularly within an intimate relationship. More subtle behavioral changes, a direct result of Masters and Johnson's work, are also occurring: women and men report, for example, a willingness for men to have intercourse and to participate in it emotionally when there is little likelihood of having an orgasm. Previously, women after orgasm would continue intercourse until the male ejaculated, but rarely vice versa. Now, if a woman feels unsatisfied some time after the male has ejaculated, they both try again even if he is but semierect. They accept the notion that offering satisfaction is not the role of only one sex.

As always, once the pendulum begins to swing, it will at times swing too far. Mr. B's experiences show how careful women must be to avoid taking over the worst of the male's definition of activity and freedom. This is no brief for the romantic sexuality espoused so strongly by Masters and Johnson in their latest book,[44] but the emotional distance and depersonalization into a "sex object" espoused by the macho cult reduces the value of human interaction when practiced by either men or women. Certainly, after all this repression, women will want to experiment and learn the old lesson anew for themselves, but perhaps they can learn from history quickly enough to avoid the worst abuses that have been practiced by men.

Judging from my unsystematic data, the chief area of experimentation to date seems to be with homosexual involvement. A number of women committed to the feminist movement who regard themselves as heterosexual feel it personally important to experience a homosexual relationship. Sometimes, this feeling results from disappointments with men, as when, in a supposedly equal relationship, the male attempts to dominate directly or indirectly. Such women want to try out a relationship unhampered by the old presumptions of sexual inferiority or superiority. Others see such a homosexual relationship as necessary to prove to themselves that they can be free of sexual dependence on men. The women I have interviewed do not intend this homosexual relationship to change their overall heterosexual orientation, but, of course, the later influence of this decision on their lives will need to be studied.

It is my impression that women who try out a homosexual affair run into less all-out concern about total sexual change than do men. In my small sample, they seem far less afraid that an experiment or two will change their overall sexual orientation. Just as men are barred from ready access to many passive responses, so a homosexual affair, past early adolescence, is terrifying for most men because it arouses powerful fears that they will be unmanned or permanently homosexual. Again, I have the impression that fears of ego dissolution rather than superego maxims are involved. One of the aims of the politically activist homosexual groups is to indicate that both men and women can be both active and passive. Being a male who is homosexually oriented need not mean that one does not function in other modes in other areas of one's life. In this aim, the homosexual groups are important pioneers for sexual egalitarianism. For the men, at least, they are trying to explore the extent to which the sexual stereotype of the lisping homosexual is another creation of the social setting. Breaking through such self-fulfilling prophecies in our society has been left to deviant groups.

Another example of some of the concerns about sex roles is the communes begun in the 1960s in the heyday of social experimentation. Most of them have had very rough going, but some of them have attempted to minimize differentiations in functioning based on sex and at times have succeeded. In trying to reach their often inchoate and overly idealistic or ideological goals, some groups experimented with group sex, both heterosexual and homosexual. In one group, the result has been the expulsion of men; the women have kept the children and are attempting to fill all roles. Another commune allots all tasks on a rotating basis, regardless of sex, and has continued to function in this fashion for seven years. Quite in contrast is the group that reacted from the rule of absolute sexual access of each to all by returning to extremely rigid sexual stereotypes, where the men work only outside the commune and the women barely leave the home. There is much to be learned from such successes and failures.

Given the extent of the misconceptions about women's capacity to function actively and passively, both sexually and productively, we are going through, and will continue for some time to go through, a period of female discovery. Inequities and disabilities resulting from those old misconceptions need to be rectified. In large measure, they have resulted from positions thoroughly accepted by our society and from the fact that the role of the social setting in affecting personality response has been little understood. If we are to prevent fresh and equally damaging misconceptions from replacing the old ones, we must remember that equality—egalitarianism—does not mean sameness. People, regardless of sex, can be equal but different. Whether at work, at home, or in the sex act, they can have different functions that are not automatically viewed as either inferior or superior.

As a result of recent research and technological changes, the harsh superego restrictions that have curtailed women's functioning will, I believe, dissolve rather quickly. As for men, however, the problems resulting from this period of social change have received little attention, mainly because of male social and sexual dominance throughout history. Yet probably a change to egalitarian sex roles will require of men a more sweeping and time-consuming reorientation of ego structure or total identity than for women. Awareness of the problem and social planning that enable men to find self-esteem and self-confidence in passive interests are necessary if these changes are to be accomplished without causing devastating social and personal disruptions.

REFERENCES

1. Friedan B: *The feminine mystique.* New York, Norton, 1963.
2. Zinberg NE: Changing stereotyped sex roles: I. Some problems for women and men, *Psychiatric Opinion* 10:25–30, 1973.
3. Zinberg NE, Jacobson RC: The natural history of "chipping," *American Journal of Psychiatry* 133:37–40, 1976.
4. Robinson P: *The modernization of sex.* New York, Harper & Row, 1976.
5. Peale E: "Normal" sex roles: An historical analysis, *Family Process* 14:389–409, 1975.
6. Thomas K: The double standard, *Journal of Social Ideas* 5:195–216, 1959.
7. Gill MM, ed.: *The collected papers of David Rapaport.* New York, Basic Books, 1967.
8. Bibring GL, Kahana RJ: *Lectures in medical psychology.* New York, International Universities Press, 1968.
9. Demos J: *A little commonwealth: Family life in Plymouth Colony.* New York, Oxford University Press, 1970.
10. Taylor GR: *The transportation revolution, 1815–1860.* New York, Harper Torchbook, 1968.
11. Graves AJ: *Women in America: Being an examination into the moral and intellectual condition in American female society.* New York, Harper & Bros., 1843.
12. deTocqueville A (1838): *Democracy in America.* Edited by Mayer JP. New York, Doubleday, 1969.
13. Grund FJ: *Aristocracy in America: From the sketchbook of a German nobleman.* New York, Harper Torchbook, 1959.
14. Zinberg NE: A return to commitment, *The Antioch Review* 26:332–344, 1966.
15. Howe I: Review of *Sexual politics,* by K. Millett, *Harper's Magazine* 241:110–125, 1970.
16. Millett K: *Sexual politics.* New York, Doubleday, 1970.

17. Strouse J, ed: *Women and analysis: Dialogues on psychoanalytic views of femininity.* New York, Dell, 1974.
18. Erikson EH: *Childhood and society.* New York, Norton, 1950.
19. Deutsch H: *The psychology of women.* (2 vols.). New York, Grune & Stratton, 1944–1945.
20. Bonaparte M: *Female sexuality.* New York, International Universities Press, 1953.
21. Lampl-de Groot J: The evolution of the Oedipus complex in women. *International Journal of Psycho-Analysis* 9:332–345, 1928.
22. Mahler MS (in collaboration with Furer M): *On human symbiosis and the vicissitudes of individuation.* New York, International Universities Press, 1968.
23. Jacobson E: *The self and the object world.* New York, International Universities Press, 1964.
24. Parsons T, Bales RF: *Family, socialization and interaction process.* Glencoe, Ill., Free Press, 1955.
25. Parsons T: Certain primary sources in patterns of aggression in the social structure of the western world, in *A study of interpersonal relations: New contributions to psychiatry.* Edited by Mullahy P. New York, Grove Press, 1957.
26. Mead M: *Male and female: A study of the sexes in a changing world.* New York, Morrow, 1949.
27. Hill GB, Powell LF, eds: *Boswell's life of Johnson.* Oxford, The Clarendon Press, 1934–1950.
28. Zinberg NE: Addiction and ego function, *Psychoanalytic Study of the Child* 30:567–598, 1975.
29. Klein GS: Psychoanalysis: II. Ego psychology, in *International Encyclopedia of the Social Sciences,* Vol. 13. Edited by Sills DL. New York, Macmillan, Free Press, 1968.
30. Jones E: *The life of Sigmund Freud,* Vol. I. New York, Basic Books, 1955.
31. Freud S (1895): Studies on hysteria. *Standard Edition* 2:3–305. London: Hogarth Press, 1955.
32. Freud S (1897): Extracts from the Fliess papers. *Standard Edition* 1:175–279. London, Hogarth Press, 1966.
33. Freud S (1930): Civilization and its discontents. *Standard Edition* 21:59–145. London, Hogarth Press, 1961.
34. Freud S (1920): Beyond the pleasure principle. *Standard Edition* 18:7–64. London, Hogarth Press, 1955.
35. Freud S (1937): Analysis terminable and interminable. *Standard Edition* 23:211–253. London, Hogarth Press, 1964.
36. Ellis HH: *Studies in the psychology of sex.* New York, Random House, 1936.
37. Krafft-Ebing Rv: *Psychopathia sexualis* (12th ed., rev. and enlarged). New York, Stein & Day, 1965.
38. Masters WH, Johnson VE: *Human sexual response.* Boston, Little, Brown, 1966.
39. Masters WH, Johnson VE: *Human sexual inadequacy.* Boston, Little, Brown, 1970.
40. Kinsey A, et al.: *Sexual behavior in the human male.* Philadelphia, W. B. Saunders, 1948.
41. Kinsey A: *Sexual behavior in the human female.* Philadelphia, W. B. Saunders, 1953.
42. Kinsey A: *The gall wasp Genus Cynips: A study in the origin of the species,* Publication #42. Bloomington, Ind., Waterman Institute for Scientific Research, 1930.
43. Kinsey A: *The origin of higher categories of Cynips.* Bloomington, Indiana University Publications, 1938.
44. Masters WH, Johnson VE: *The pleasure bond: A new look at sexuality and commitment.* Boston, Little, Brown, 1974.
45. *Mike Nichols and Elaine May Examine Doctors.* Mercury Records, #20680. 1968.

46. Ginsberg GL, Frosch WA, Shapiro T: The new impotence. *Archives of General Psychiatry 26*:218–220, 1972.
47. Bowlby J: *Separation: Anxiety and anger.* London, Hogarth Press, 1973.
48. Klein M: *Envy and gratitude: A study of unconscious sources.* London, Tavistock, 1957.
49. Kohut H: *The analysis of the self.* New York, International Universities Press, 1971.
50. Spitz R: *The first year of life.* New York, International Universities Press, 1971.
51. Winnicott DW: *The maturational processes and the facilitating environment.* London, Hogarth Press, 1965.
52. Rapaport D: *The structure of psychoanalytic theory.* New York, International Universities Press, 1960.
53. Gill MM, Brenman M: *Hypnosis and related states.* New York, International Universities Press, 1959.
54. Hartmann H (1939): *Ego psychology and the problem of adaptation.* New York, International Universities Press, 1958.
55. Klein GS: Consciousness in psychoanalytic theory: Some implications for current research in perception, *Journal of the American Psychoanalytic Association 7*:5–34, 1959.
56. Orwell G: *1984.* New York: Harcourt Brace, 1949.
57. Zinberg NE: *"High"* states: A beginning study, Drug Abuse Council Publication SS-3. Washington, D.C.: Drug Abuse Council, 1974.
58. Skinner BF: *Walden two.* New York, Macmillan, 1948.

Chapter 4

The Black Woman Growing Up

VEVA H. ZIMMERMAN

George Segal,[1] in a painterly reflection on mood, addressed his near obsession with human identity, saying, "I could establish an identity in solid plaster, but could make it slide by changing colors. By choosing different colors I can run the gamut of the way I feel." Therein he also touched the haunting theme in the developing self-image of a black woman, where the feature of color clouds all the rest in its importance in identity formation. Skin color inherently carries a complex social meaning for both observer and owner. Yet, what Segal has cogently depicted in his technique is the very *separateness* of person and color.

The black person has come to expect in each new encounter with whites because of skin color that she* will be arbitrarily assigned an identity that is stereotypically derived from the white person's image of a "black person." This image has a stranglehold on the minds of white persons in this society and is perpetuated by the social separation between the majority of the members of the two groups despite major achievements in the advance toward the integration of educational services during the past 20 years.

Any consideration of postadolescent development in a black woman must begin in that central focus of personal skin color, for it brings a series of problems, benefits, and needs that must be comfortably integrated into the individual's picture of herself. This task must be completed before a successful resolution of the common quest for

---

*The feminine pronouns are used here because of the format of the book, but this information is applicable to males as well.

VEVA H. ZIMMERMAN, M.D. ● Department of Psychiatry, New York University School of Medicine, New York.

intimacy, freedom to work, and capacity for healthy self-esteem, seen universally in postadolescent identity, can take place.

The adolescent generally has struggled with establishing, once and for all, a separate self beyond the definition of the family and of extra-familial relationships. She has hopefully emerged from those battles with parents and from her own fears of personal inadequacy with a workable definition of herself as a daughter, as a student or a worker, a lover, a spouse, or even a parent. During the late teens and early 20s, she will make even further strides toward autonomy if all goes well for her in finding her own family, friends, work, and social nexus.

Postadolescence is then an amorphous period between adolescence proper and young adulthood, which is not delineated by age so much as by psychological issues. The central task of adolescence and postadolescence is the formation of a relatively stable sense of identity, which is usually achieved in parallel with psychological separation from the parents.

The postadolescent, usually in her early to mid-20s, has to function much more independently now than ever before. The sense of herself that she has developed during late adolescence is now put through the test of how well it holds up without the protections provided during those earlier years from family and school.

Her sense of self is modified, supported, or threatened by how successful she is in meeting reality's demands. This sense of identity, then, is not merely a static internal image. It develops largely out of interactions with others and is altered through time as a result of feedback from others, as well as from one's own observing ego and superego. It contains the various roles one has to "perform" and learn, for example, sex roles and professional roles. The development of the sense of a self capable of relatively stable, successful, independent functioning is the hoped-for outcome of postadolescence.

Of course, what is "successful" depends on a realistic evaluation of one's abilities and the related modification of one's ego ideal so that internal expectations are not grandiose or unrealistic. This reality testing and modification of the ego ideal, which normally has its beginnings in early childhood and continues through adolescence, is a *crucial* task for the postadolescent establishing a place in a dual society. The failure to establish this process can result in such symptoms as dysphoria, depression, chronic feelings of failure, and/or boredom. The maintenance of self-esteem is facilitated if one's ideals and expectations are realistic and if one is successfully able to meet these internal standards and demands. While the need for positive feedback from others certainly continues to exist, by the end of postadolescence the main source of self-esteem should be satisfaction with one's self based on internalized standards. Only then is the healthy independence of maturity possible.

THE BLACK WOMAN

During postadolescence, the black woman must come to some resolution of her own racial conflicts. She must achieve a workable definition of herself in her various roles in an essentially white society, without violating her sense of blackness, in order to provide for the maintenance of self-esteem and a feeling of personal adequacy. This achievement is difficult in our society, because of the pervasive rejection of blackness as undesirable.

The resolution of this status issue requires learning the intricate social skills needed to find an effective voice in one's out-group role; it also requires learning skills that preserve one's personal sense of blackness intact and as noninterfering. This kind of learning demands the effective resolution of conflict stemming from being angry at society. It demands the learning of respect for other individuals, both in-group and out, even when one feels threatened with rejection. It means developing comfort in dealing with assertive issues with other people, especially if those relationships are with whites. Blacks who live in integrated settings during adolescence may evade situations that require aggression or assertiveness. They may isolate themselves by restricting themselves, out of anxiety, to their own racial group, or they may fail to approach the people they need assistance from at school, on jobs, etc., compounding their sense of isolation.

Unconscious reactions to being an object of racial prejudice can result in exactly the same symptom formation as is produced by early fears of irrational reprisals from powerful parents, namely, direct inhibition with substitutive object displacement and inept modulation of affect. For example, a student found it impossible to relate to the graduate school faculty where she was studying. When she first arrived, she was able to speak up in lectures and to ask questions. During the first year, she became increasingly withdrawn, spending most of her time with a black man in her class who was academically successful. Her performance progressively deteriorated. Behind this withdrawal was an acute sensitivity, which made her feel that she was unwanted at the school, misinterpreting the institutional behavior that everyone is subject to, like lost applications. The more withdrawn she became, the poorer a student she became, and the more her sense of not belonging increased, the greater her failure.

MANAGEMENT OF ANGER

The special task that minority women encounter through the course of their adolescent and postadolescent development is the achievement of an important cohesion incorporating a stable core image of the self that is at once acceptable to its owner and yet functional in the society. This task is, of course, set for everyone, but the specific ways in which this process is disrupted by racial experiences are numerous:

1. Vigilance about trusting others not to prejudge, or misjudge, is constant, rendering it difficult for the young person to maneuver comfortably outside an immediate social group. In short, defending oneself against stereotyping is an experience akin to having one's personality and character assessed on the single basis of one's wearing an occupational uniform (e.g., as a nurse, a policeman, or a sanitation worker).

The black youth's behavior often becomes stereotyped or reactive in a predetermined manner.

2. The American black is angry much of the time. This anger is often not directly observable, but it is nonetheless there. The sociologist Powdermaker[2] has very nicely enumerated the various pathways that American blacks can be observed to follow in handling aggression within the society. These are:

a. Direct aggression (highly unusual before the late 1960s).
b. Displacement onto other blacks.
c. Retreat into the "ivory tower," for example, by an essential denial of the problem's effect on one's own life.
d. Identification with the white mentor or employer.
e. Diversion of aggression into wit.
f. Meek, humble, nonaggressive black deference to whites, no matter what the provocation (e.g., the "Uncle Tom" figure).

Behind this latter solution is the important observation that the suppression of affect is conscious. When whites are not around, the stronger personality tone emerges in the company of other blacks. There is pleasure in the secrecy and the sense of putting something over on the "enemy."

3. In American culture, the perception of difference is often a hostile event that pursues interrelationships, as with blacks, wherever it occurs; this negative perception is accepted by the black and the white. Hence, the specter of rejection of what may be prized in the self is a constant threat for the black woman. This negative perception also correlates with social and economic class differences, which often further delineate the ethnic groups. For instance, let's examine the med-

ical school setting, since many of the people discussed in this paper are medical or graduate students. In medical school, the average white student comes from a comfortable, middle-class or professional-class home, whereas the average black student comes from a lower-middle-class home, comfortable but not in the same style as the more affluent white group. These class differences are further reflected in differences in the spending money available, the use of vacation time, attitudes toward low-income patients, and rapport with the maintenance personnel in the medical center.

Nonblacks commonly fail to distinguish socioeconomic differences between blacks; hence, a black medical student commonly will be mistakenly addressed as the orderly or the cleaning woman on the ward by patients and visitors, something that generates further anger in the black.

Studies in psychology, sociology, and psychiatry (Eugene Brody,[3,4] Kenneth Clark,[5] and M. McDonald[6]) provide insights into the almost universal American opinion of blackness as inferior and undesirable observable in black and white children. Other studies (e.g., Hauser[7]) imply that identity resolution is altered in some way for black youths. The anger generated in American blacks because of the social caste system has been poignantly explored in the novel and in dramatic literature.

Black adolescents living in but not raised in an integrated society routinely have two social personalities, one for predominantly black-dominated groups and one for nonblack groups. This distinction often persists into later life. From my own experience, when I would ride the elevators at Bellevue, a black woman doctor in mixed company, the black employees would be subdued. If there were no white professional staff or visitors on the car, the black workers would joke and speak without restraint in a more natural "black" tone and manner, with body language, humor, and "color." When I was around, I was never directly, but always tacitly, included in their somewhat distant friendliness.

These different roles can easily lead to a more serious and pathological split in identity. Blacks sensitive to this development in themselves often comment on experiencing an "emptiness" when in the company of blacks alone, as if their primary strivings are toward the "white" style. In contrast, blacks leaning toward the "black" style feel subtly hostile, disturbed, and constricted in mixed company. When blacks are alone with whites, they may enjoy a kind of "special" status that alleviates the sense of alienation and modifies their manner. One or the other resolution of this conflict is hard to avoid, even with the obvious pitfalls attached to either choice. If one chooses the "white" style, one could be rejecting one's racial identity as black. If one chooses the "black" style, one largely rejects the possibility of positive interaction with white groups, which can greatly restrict opportunities for personal and professional interaction and development. Black middle-class postadolescents seeking to enter professions and white-collar jobs cannot really avoid this dilemma.

As a result of racial prejudice and the caste system, which continues to exist in our society, the black adolescent is far more burdened than is her white peer with the struggle to be regarded by others as an individual rather than a stereotype. This conflict over individual treatment versus stereotyping occurs not just in relating to whites but also in relating to other blacks, because of the once-prominent emphasis on skin shading in black social and family groups. This emphasis, fortunately, is currently diminishing. Often, each new relationship, whether with a black or a white, brings up the question of whether this new person is going to relate to the individual for her own qualities or first as a black person, including the assignment of admired qualities as well as critical ones. For instance, in the integrated group, the black woman is often seen as special when she has attributes like warmth, competence, and understanding. The white woman in the same group with similar qualities would probably not be as highly regarded. The black woman may understandably respond to this high regard as a personal compliment, but often underneath is the nagging reality of the subtle assignment of increased value to the desirable traits in the black woman because of the feeling that most of the black group are different, with decreased value. Such an example is the common myth that a black student in medical school got there by privilege, not merit.*

INTERACTING WITH OTHERS

There is a kind of void that is marked, in the life of the individual, by social and political circumstances beyond her control. Let's look at the interchange between a black patient and a white professional as a limited but illustrative example of the cognitive dissonance set up by stereotyping (Table 1).

These two will never make an effective pair in health-care deliv-

---

*It is not clear whether this bias stems from the increased numbers of economically disadvantaged blacks in white schools or is due more to the prevalent federal and Association of American Medical Colleges' efforts to increase black and Hispanic enrollment in the late 1960s. Prior to that time, the lone black in the class would be seen as "superbright."

Table I. Analysis of the Doctor–Patient Interchange

White or black doctor, middle-class	Black patient, middle-class
1. Achievement-oriented.	2. Wants information and/or aid.
3. Awareness of subject's blackness—wishes to demonstrate special sympathetic interests.	4. Awareness of race, white or black, wants to be heard individually, not as a representative of collective experience.
5. Feels slightly rebuffed, tries harder.	6. Feels reaffirmed about being idealized or romanticized, hence ignored as an individual.
7. Feels puzzled and flounders.	8. Feels hostile and sullen or turned off.
9. Reasserts authority of role to demand cooperation.	10. Rejects authority of doctor's role and feels secretly superior/inadequate and convinced of the other's racism or Uncle Tomism.

ery. Neither can hear the other; yet neither is guilty of the so-called traditional concept of racism, that of caste assignment with hostile segregation. It is caste assignment with the more subtle twists of paternalism.

The most important lesson for both individuals to learn is to focus on the common task. Patience, with enough flexibility from a healthy self-concept, can guide the misguided doctor back to the task of diagnosis or treatment. The doctor must resist being overly interested in the patient's blackness and must start with the data needed, thus keeping the work focused and establishing a viable bond between them that allows a maximum of self-respect. The doctor should do what the doctor knows best, diagnosing illness; the patient should provide the necessary information and cooperation to get the relief or the answer sought. People can often tolerate not being loved, but failing to gain a minimum of respect is more difficult to tolerate.

In some ways, the experience of the black is parallel to the experience of the disabled. The polio victim enters a room full of partying people. She wants to be noticed as a person, but instead, because of the natural drift of human curiosity toward the disabled, she is usually seen first as a person limping. Much enlightened consciousness-raising has been brought to bear on the general public to overlook the limp, or the scarred mask of the burn survivor, or the notch of the harelip child. The crippled child has been bolstered and told that idle curiosity is rudeness and human thoughtlessness, not a devaluation of her own character. Hence, both sides in this drama have often had some preparation on these issues prior to the paralytic's entry into the crowded room. The stronger child learns this formulation and bulldozes forward, keeping her mind on meeting others, like the terrified actress who has learned to worry about what the role needs, rather than her own visibility.

In fitting contrast, civil activism has roused the guilt and shame of large groups of liberally disposed professionals and has stimulated their wish to correct the unfairness and to affirmatively demonstrate their willingness to "like" the black. The black isn't interested primarily in being liked as a black but is concerned about getting medical care, and then, secondarily, about being accepted and not rejected. She should be concerned about not becoming rejecting, in turn.

VIEW OF FAMILY RELATIONS

The young child needs a period of relatively unqualified approval from objects whom she respects until her own basic sense of worth and of her importance to others is firmly internalized. The black child is often blessed with warm familial relationships that nurture her before her exposure to the outside color bias, but often, in early childhood, usually about the time of her entry into school, she discovers that the family lives with a compromised image in the outside world. In addition, black families, particularly those from the middle class, are often tough, especially on black girls, wanting them to stay sheltered at home.

Freud, in *The Interpretation of Dreams,*[8] tells of the experience of feeling humiliation for his father when, as they walked together in Vienna, his father stepped in the gutter to let a gentile pass.

These following experiences carry out the same theme that Freud described.

> A highly intelligent and sensitive black woman working as a patient in psychotherapy was struggling to accept herself as the accomplished educator she had become, when she recalled a vivid image of her father as impotent in his conflict with a sheriff who presumptively arrested him as the black on the scene without justifiable evidence of his guilt, and of her guilt as she recalled that she had struggled to decide who was right, the sheriff or her father, who denied the charge.

> Another black woman, the daughter of a surgeon, experienced confusion and shame when she watched her much-admired, successful, and usually aggressive father walk away from two hillbillies who had injured her companion. She and the daughter of her father's office nurse were in the rear seat of the car at a gas station. The adults had left the car to attend to errands, leaving word for the girls not to get out of the car. The two

men were sitting near the gas pumps and called the girls. The other child disobeyed and went to see what they wanted. One suddenly grabbed her by the neck and held her up, stretching her cervical spine to the point of severe pain.

Another medical student's world at home had been one of physics and philosophy problems, spoken of and played over with authority around the dining-room table. There, her father was the benevolent ruler of the household. Outside, he was a Pullman porter, and his daughter played with the children of prostitutes and petty criminals on the stoop.

The faces of ghetto youngsters often change during second and third grade from open, alert, good-humored expressions to solemn, duller ones. The normal childhood idealization of the parents has been brought into question prematurely, before the child has developed the basis for an internalized sense of worth.

At this critical moment, the child can either lose respect for her parent, which leaves her own self-esteem too vulnerable to society's disapproval and rejection; or she can adopt the protective pseudomature role of being dedicated to protecting the parent and rectifying the social ill. This latter route can foster relative quiet during the skill-learning periods of latency and adolescence, and the child can achieve a surface success in academics, peer relations, interracial socializing, etc. However, as a consequence of this premature and defensive development of a sense of self-worth, the underlying confusion often reemerges with divisive results when the individual is trying to integrate a self-image in the early 20s—when trying to get married, graduate, achieve commitment to work, and enter a profession, especially when role playing is important or the child can experience racial ambiguity and personal confusion.

Mattie, a student in her third year of college, began to experience periods of apathy and confusion. She was very experienced in integrated settings. Her first placement had been in an integrated nursery school at age 4, and she continued in integrated schools from there on through college.

She was sent to a camp where she was the only black child enrolled. During this period she began to experience feelings that she was white. These feelings did not involve the negation of blacks and are a common experience among blacks who are essentially alone in large white groups from early ages. Her skin was not as visible to her as to someone else.* She was continuously in the position of looking at skin that was nonblack rather than being aware of her own color; hence, it was easier for her to feel like those around her, and she was rapidly assimilated into the group. Her family's attitudes toward blacks were friendly, but they did not socialize actively with blacks or whites. More importantly, their educational priori-

*Striking support for the supposition that visible evidence of skin color is a singularly influential characteristic.

ties were parallel to those of the white group and different from those of
many of the blacks whom they knew.

When this student was faced with choosing a career, the old solution
became exposed and threatened her. She did apply to medical school, was
accepted, and successfully performed the first two years, but far below her
potential level of achievement.

Social skills that are developed by successful blacks, and that are
acceptable to the black group as well as to whites, closely parallel general, healthy ego development, with special emphasis on the skills listed
in Table 2.

This table is a partial listing of the ego tasks that are involved.
When the woman fails to master a significant number of these skills,
certain "racial" conflicts develop.

These conflicts may become manifest as difficulty asserting herself
in work or social situations; fear of dealing with issues in depth, resulting in superficiality; or revulsion toward her own racial group,
leading to haughtiness. One patient with an obsessive-compulsive
neurosis constantly complained about examples of this same behavior
in peers of black-oriented groups, out of fear of these same failings in
herself. Inner confusion is common in this age group. Sometimes, it
is hidden behind an apparent paralysis, which seems to be due to
neurotic inhibition. Sometimes, it is hidden behind an intense commitment to the tenets of "black supremacy," which may lead to bitterness, cynicism, or reverse racism. It is important to separate these
manifestations from a healthy expression of racial advocacy and pride.

Table II. Ego Function and Personality Development

Critical skills	Important but less critical skills
1. Self-recognition.	1. Pride, both self and racial.
2. Conceptual growth.	2. Self-image as professional, etc.
3. Maintenance of self-esteem in the face of failure, guilt, or other noxious experience.	3. Self as feminine.
4. Managing anger.	4. Comfortable late family relations.
5. Healthy early family relationships.	5. Self as spouse, confidante, etc.
6. Peer involvements: respect for others and social skills, including handling racial situations.	6. Insight into distorted demands on society, such as guilt or rage.
7. Recognition of racism, technique of management of perception of others and reactivity to others.	
8. Development of social ideals.	

The differentiating features are usually similar to the general signs of maturity, for example, signs of ego integrity, flexibility, and the ability to relate to others, to maintain self-esteem, to grow, and to work in a reasonable manner. Those individuals with an unresolved conflict are prone to difficulties in establishing relationships with others, peers and authority figures alike. The black woman may buy the racial stereotype—for example, "disadvantaged students"—but at an unconscious level, then in anger act this out or react against it.

> A young resident recalled being confronted by an attending physician who asked whether she knew some elementary information from her discipline. She knew she did but said, "No!" He persisted, "Do you not know or are you afraid to tell me?" She repeated, "No! I don't know," aware that she was lying. Her consciousness dimly brushed by the fleeting thought, "He doesn't think I know anyway." As she explained her behavior years later, she went on to explain that she assumed that he, knowing she was black, would automatically assume that she was ignorant, unlike her fellow white residents. She thought this despite her conscious realistic experience with this supervisor as someone who sometimes respected her work.

Another story illustrates the group behavior that perpetuates this pejorative racial image:

> In 1974, a flash rumor spread among the black medical students at two medical colleges in New York City, that an instructor in a basic science course at a third medical school had openly said to a group of black students in the first-year class who were having academic troubles, "We will send you back to the kitchen where you belong." This rumor was accepted by those who heard it. One student who internalized this incident became increasingly depressed about striving to join a "white" profession and ended up failing the first part of her National Board exams, a licensing procedure, even though her grades in the same subjects in her school exams had been good. Her conflict boiled down to "I am leaving my group to become a doctor—I will become white, I will reject my blackness."

This group identified itself as much by the egregious slander as by its own real accomplishments.

> Another young woman nearly destroyed her chances to finish medical school by cutting labs and being hostile and sullen to her preclinical instructors, who, despite her standoffishness and apparent lack of interest, picked up that she was exceptionally talented. She failed her exams because she did not study the material. She then was given the choice of repeating the exams or repeating the year. At that point, she became suicidally depressed. Emergency psychotherapy was begun. What emerged was that she was failing in a relationship with her boyfriend, who was clearly threatened by her intellectual gifts. Because of a similar relationship with her brother, who also lost family status because he had less intellectual skill, she was trapped into believing she would never be married if she were bright. The solution was not to finish medical school. She did not seem to respond to the comment made by the therapist that she seemed

to feel the old stereotype that women who are bright can't make it. What released her ability to study for the makeup exam and pass it with a high grade was becoming aware of her own fantasized belief that black men aren't smart but are usually outstripped by black women.

Another young woman, a graduate student in social work, impressed the faculty as exceptionally bright, but she was unable to function academically. She cut classes, was tardy in assignments, and refused to participate in discussions. In psychotherapy, improvement followed a brief confrontation with the acting-out character of her behavior when she demonstrated it in the transference relationship with her therapist. She was also helped by the effect of role modeling, since the therapist was clearly black and was functioning successfully in a white community.

Many of these issues affect black male and female adolescents alike. The constriction in performance described above can become manifest as an inability to potentiate a talent for learning science.

A shy but extremely bright young student entered medical school with a strong interest in neuroscience research. She had already had some experience, so it was easy for her to obtain work in a lab at the school. During her second year, she developed conversion symptoms and was unable to ask questions in either lectures or seminars. She would start to speak after raising her hand, only to find that she could not speak. Only squeaks would come out because of a laryngospasm.

The inhibition disappeared in five psychotherapy sessions, after she became aware that she felt that her fellow minority students thought her too "intellectual." This fantasy developed in the middle of a guilty rage at her father, who was demanding the right to drop into the dormitory on unannounced visits to chat with his daughter. The father clearly was proud of his daughter but was unable to grasp and respond to the student's genuine quandary over the time lost by such visits. The overt rejection activated guilt over a much subtler rejection of the father's unschooled interests and traditional authoritarian, patriarchial style. This style contrasted painfully, for the student, with the camaraderie of the white faculty father-figures whom she had come to admire at the Ivy League school she attended. This style is so clearly "white," that wanting such experiences with a white and not a black equaled rejection of the black. She further felt that other minority students perceived her "prejudice" and, in turn, would reject her, and so she reacted symptomatically to hide her intellectual proclivity. This complicated, convoluted issue completely impaired her image in seminars and made her look shy and unable to follow the material. Once the symptom occurred, she was too embarrassed even to attempt to speak to the instructor after class. We see the contrapuntal theme of racial conflict within a common parent–child scenario.

Young adults who have grown up in integrated settings, where there is little opportunity for the black child to experience the comfortable acceptance of her own racial group, give histories that suggest that the stereotyping they endured as children will lead to important disturbances in character formation and subtle disturbances in affectual adjustment to social situations in adulthood. These individuals are prone to chronically low self-esteem. A significant number of them appear chronically depressed. Problems commonly occur when a black family, in an effort to gain opportunities for superior education for their children, place a child in an integrated classroom where she is the sole black child.

> Mattie (previously discussed) was started on this path as a nursery-school student after four years of contacts with only black peers. She managed well during those years, made friends, performed well, and developed musical talents, gaining extra recognition for these. However, in college, she felt overwhelmed by conflict with the socially aware, outspoken blacks of the early 1970s at the prestigious Ivy League school she attended. She managed to do well enough to get into a good medical school, but she slipped rapidly into a state of confusion, social withdrawal, obesity, and depression that impaired her ability to give medicine more than the cursory attention required to pass.
>
> The banter of these outspoken students opened up an anxious, conflicted experience for this student. She became so confused about who she was that she was unable to proceed to acquire any new identity. The professionalization stressed in medical school drives the student toward assuming the group character of "physician." This student was unable to assume a "medical student's image" because of her unclear racial identity. Instead, she went around severely confused and in a state of apathy.
>
> Another student was moved to second grade in a neighboring suburb as soon as the schools there opened to blacks. At the point when that system became more integrated because of newly arriving blacks, her mother moved her into a private secondary school, where again she was the lone black in her class. She always did moderately well in her studies, but her personality functioning carried the aura of a person walking with heavy ankle counterweights in deep water. She was chronically depressed and was often described by her colleagues as "the most inhibited individual" they'd met. She improved after she was able to see herself master the work in medical school.

SUMMARY

These stories chronicle the latent pain and confusion that continue to haunt the black children of this society, even those considered liberated by their gifts of talent, intelligence, and inner sophistication in comparison with the less fortunate black peers from their high schools. These youths, for the most part, will succeed in the world, with degrees and occupations that surpass what fate seemed to have in store for them, but at an enormous price.

None of the observations contained in these vignettes are unusual, and all have been made in other groups. The difference lies in the pervasive influence of the experience. Most important is the underlying dilemma that faces these individuals. If they join the mainstream of society, they risk the loss of that part of the self that includes the racial self. If they reject the society in which they live, they cut themselves off from the fruits of their efforts. The best solutions clearly lie in integration. Yet, it is impossible for any American black to forget the haunting image of the "undesirable black." Because of the long history of the caste system in this country, these individuals have little support from group pride from within the black community. This circumstance, too, is changing, so that blacks in this country are learning to support their successful members, but at this writing, this experience is true only for isolated individuals.

Baldwin[9] and Lacy[10] have presented an eloquent description of people searching to find themselves in the wake of the suppression and the confusion imposed by unremitting anger. They, as well as Morrison,[11] have described some of the more contorted personal solutions adopted by individual blacks in order to function in the face of this anger.

Behind these comments, there are special young women from whom I have had the privilege of learning much about their private lives. There are many illustrations from other young men and women whom I know well for varied professional reasons, as psychiatrist, as counselor to medical students both for personal distress and academic problems, and as colleague or co-worker. In the core group, all have managed to develop admirable careers in medicine, or psychology, or social work, or business. A striking number of similarities can be found in each of their lives. They are all angry, but often mask their anger with argumentative, vigorous good humor, which lends support to their successful adjustment as significant spokespeople for their student groups. Each of these people has experienced significant depression. Some writers[12] have suggested that blacks have less vulnerability to serious depressive states, because of the potential opportunity to project guilt onto external objects, such as society at large. My experience does not support this suggestion. The depression is universal; only the style of expression is different.[13] Often, it is much less visible because of the tendency for blacks who are depressed to manifest their depression as depressive equivalent symptoms, such as by negativism, diffidence mixed with a flamboyant personal style, or, as expressed by another individual, a near-paranoid retreat into the dialectics of the racism that destroys his or her ability to recognize the individuals in the faculty whom he or she has to deal with and to see the problem only as a global one. Many of this group show social aloofness and periodic behavioral disturbances. Some suffer from cynical disaffection from the school, their own career goals, and their own family members. Even two of the healthiest have an officiousness in their manner that increases social distance and prevents heterosexual success.

This paper is an attempt to explore the development of self-esteem in the postadolescent black woman in a manner that highlights the potential disruptions in development caused by the peculiar structure of the racial caste system in American black–white relations. Comfortable access to assertive behavior must be present in each individual to preserve her potential to influence other people and to gain a rightful place in society. It cannot be forgotten that assertion is an inner psychic experience that is frequently associated with conflict. The black woman is faced with external inhibitions as well, deriving from the society in which she lives. Black anger is a provocative state. When it becomes externally visible, it may provoke responsive suspicion or fear in the surrounding group that is unwarranted by the true intensity of the particular black individual's feeling or motives. All of these conflicts, internal and external, may seriously interfere with life goals by creating inhibition or by interfering with the perception of the signals from the environment. They may also lead to distortions in interpreting society's responses.

Not all anger is bad. Self-righteous, nonguilty, object-directed, appropriate anger is often clarifying and healthy. The angry child who responds to real stimuli generally grows up to be more resistant to external pressure than the passive, compliant child, who often is forced to give up a significant picture of herself in order to survive.

In the striving black individual, resentment can interfere with the individual's learning professionally or can provoke cynical withdrawal in a situation where significant learning comes from relationships with colleagues. These mechanisms often interfere with flexible responsivity to peers and friends from nonblack groups.

The racial stereotyping that is extremely common in daily American life has important intrapsychic effects on the black woman's development. The development of acceptable beauty standards, for example, affects the black woman's image of herself. Her choice of standards of social behavior and of intellectual and occupational interests may threaten to alienate her from the black group, and her skin color stands as a permanent testimony to her difference from the white society. This one feature evokes a predetermined set of images and reactions that can be indiscriminately applied. The black woman constantly faces this potential judgmental alienation. The 1960s and 1970s have brought increased sophistication, but stereotyping remains. The automatic identification of a given individual with a group of disparaged individuals is the offshoot of the old caste system, and the rigid

definition of this group leads to the "annihilation of the self," the
enigma of the black woman growing up.

REFERENCES

1. Segal G: Sculpture Exhibition, Whitney Museum, New York, 1979.
2. Powdermaker H: The channeling of Negro aggression by the cultural process, in *Personality in nature, society and culture* (2nd ed.). Edited by Kluckhohn C, Murray HA. New York, Knopf, 1953.
3. Brody EB: Color and identity conflict in young boys: Observations of Negro mothers and sons in urban Baltimore, *Psychiatry* 26 (2):188–201, May 1963.
4. Brody EB: Color and identity conflict in young boys. II: Observations of white mothers and sons in urban Baltimore. *Archives of General Psychiatry* April 10, 1964, 354–360.
5. Clark K: *Prejudice and your child* (2nd ed.). Boston, Beacon Press, 1963.
6. McDonald M: *Not by the color of their skin*. New York, International Universities Press, 1970.
7. Hauser ST: Black and white identity development: Aspects and perspectives, *Journal of Youth and Adolescence* 1 (2):113–130, 1972.
8. Freud S: *The interpretation of dreams*. New York, Science Editions, 1961.
9. Baldwin J: *Notes of a native son*. Boston, Beacon Press, 1955.
10. Lacy LA: *The rise and fall of a proper Negro: An autobiography*. New York, Macmillan, 1970.
11. Morrison T: *Song of Solomon*. New York, Knopf, 1977.
12. Prange A, Vitols M: Cultural aspects of the relatively low incidence of depression in Southern Negroes. *International Journal of Soc. Psychiatry* 8:104–112, 1962.
13. Halpern F: Personal communication. 1976

SUPPLEMENTARY READING

Brickner RP: *My second twenty years: An unexpected life*. New York, Basic Books, 1976.
Erikson EH: *Childhood and society*. New York, Norton, 1950.
Erikson EH: *Identity, youth and crisis*. New York, Norton, 1968.
Halpern F: *Survival black/white*. New York, Pergamon Press, 1973.
King SH: *Five lives at Harvard: Personality change during college*. Cambridge, Mass., Harvard University Press, 1973.
Kolb L: The role of identification in the achievement of goals, The working papers of the 1975 Conference on Education of Psychiatrists. Edited by Busse E, Sussex JN. American Psychiatric Association, 1976.
Kvaraceus WC, Gibson TS, Patterson FK, Seasholes B, Grambs JD: *Negro self-concept implications for school and citizenship*. New York, McGraw-Hill, 1965.
Paykel E, *et al*: Treatment setting and clinical depression, *Archives of General Psychiatry* 22 (1):1–21, 1970.
Persell CH: *Education and inequality*. New York, Free Press, 1977.
Powell GJ: *Black Mondays children*. New York, Appleton-Century-Crofts, 1973.
Wittenberg R: *Postadolescence, theoretical and clinical aspects of psychoanalytic therapy*. New York, Grune & Stratton, 1968.

PART II

Life Cycle Considerations

Chapter 5

The Early Mother–Child Relationship: A Developmental View of Woman as Mother

T. BERRY BRAZELTON AND CONSTANCE H. KEEFER

> *Every signal which establishes a new premise or pact bringing the persons closer together or giving them greater freedom may be a source of joy. But every signal which falls by the wayside is in some degree a source of pain to both.*
> GREGORY BATESON, *The Natural History of an Interview*, 1971

The process of becoming a mother is a complex developmental sequence involving a search for a particular identity as a woman. Helene Deutsch gave us a framework for understanding this process. She pointed out its biological and psychological nature and the unique experience it provides, "in which a woman is given the opportunity of experiencing a real sense of immortality and of the victory of life over death." [1] The successful search means a movement from the diffusion of youth to the completeness and reality of adulthood. Interrelationships between the mother and her child, her mate, and her parents must undergo expansion and clarification. Success in this process is made possible by the fact that these relationships, particularly that with her child, will fuel the mother's own growth.

A specific focus of this growth process is "how to mother," and this is truly a struggle for women today. They turn to us as professionals, and in the process, we see their anguish and caring. Their efforts at maturing and nurturing are not supported, and we often see their caring devalued.

Our particular role, that of pediatricians dedicated to the mainte-

T. BERRY BRAZELTON, M.D., AND CONSTANCE H. KEEFER, M.D. • Children's Hospital Medical Center, Harvard Medical School, Boston, Massachusetts. This paper was written under the support of the Robert Wood Johnson Foundation, Princeton, New Jersey.

nance of the physical and emotional growth of children, has placed us in a special relationship to these mothers. It is a dual relationship, one in which the mother is our ally with the child in her care, and one in which we can seek out and support the mother's feelings and concerns about the child, and her interactions with the child become a focus for our attention.

We have therefore been allowed to observe women going through this struggle to become mothers. These observations have led us to a developmental view of this struggle, and we see how it pertains to the mother's developing relationship with her infant. We see it as a major growth opportunity for women and a potentially positive one for most of them. An understanding of the development of mothering, therefore, becomes an important tool for any professional to whom mothers turn for help.

Our focus on mothers in this paper results from our clinical contacts and research efforts with them. It does not imply that fathers' relationships with their children are not equally significant to the mother–infant relationship or equally relevant to the mother's development. Fathering has not been the subject of such critical research as mothering, and our clinical contacts with fathers are for the most part too few to have led to a conceptualization of a developmental process. (The fact that fathers have not been the focus of concern or investigation is perhaps a demonstration of the ambivalence and confusion about parenting in our society.) Where possible, we draw here on the clinical impressions we have and on the relevant research available to highlight the unique aspects of father–infant relationships and their effects on the mother–infant relationship.

At this point, it is possible to say that, aside from the specific effects of the father–infant relationship, a supportive relationship between mother and father allows the mother more security and more flexibility in her role, and a protected sphere within which she can safely explore and experiment with her relationship with her child.

The mother's dependency on professionals and the need for appropriate responses to it are particularly acute today for a number of reasons. The small nuclear family, mobile and distant from whatever extended family may exist, is the framework within which many women become mothers. This phenomenon allows for little support for young mothers from a more experienced generation. The problem is only exacerbated by the fact that the isolation of the nuclear family is not just physical and geographical but is part of an emotional stratification and separation of generations as well.[2] Thus, the young mother is unable to turn to her own mother for help when she needs her.

The nuclear family has been the model for so long that many of the women who are now becoming mothers have come from small nuclear families themselves. A result of this historical decline in the extended family is a loss of the important experience of observing and being involved in the care of infants as a child oneself.

A young woman today, therefore, has had no early experience with children and has no built-in family supports to assist her in developing her role as mother. The course many women take is to turn to professionals, who are presumed to have more understanding than the young mother of childhood and mothering. The intensity with which young mothers latch on to professionals who have an interest in children or women is a reflection of how great their need is and of how much they care about their children and their roles as mothers. It should not be taken to mean that professional input is necessary to carry out that role. We could look to many more effective sources of support than can be provided by such professionals. But at present, these sources are not available, and pediatricians and nurse practitioners may be. What is needed first is professional understanding of the important positive aspects of the role, as well as sanction of and support for a woman's independent development in it. Second, professionals must work toward changing some of the negative, devaluating attitudes of society toward the role. There are three such attitudes that are particularly prevalent and seem destructive.

The first is that society is ambivalent with regard to the tangible values placed on the role of mothering. While motherhood is classically given an exalted position in American society, this has been so only in terms of a one-sided giving relationship, tied to a homemaking service, and exclusive of other creative aspects. When measured by any available objective standard for "success," this role falls short. This has become clear in a study carried out by the second author in which the experiences of women with professional careers, having their first babies, were examined. These women all had a clear sense of their value in society regarding their professional roles. When they became mothers, they found no similar confirmation of the value of their roles as mothers. In fact, they continued to have that role measured by the standards of their professional roles (e.g., efficiency, income production, power, and ripple effect), and in that comparison, they fell short.

The second destructive message comes from a competitive standard applied to child rearing. This leads to an expectation of "perfect mother—perfect child," an impossible goal. The message is that the baby will be molded directly by her or his mother (without any contribution on the child's part or any sense of interaction). Therefore, young mothers are forced to walk a tightrope of total responsibility, with failure imminent on either side: whatever the mother does to the child is likely to lead to irreversible psychopathology in the child's future; whatever she doesn't do for the child will lead to cognitive impairment in the child and school failure. Unfortunately, in many situations, even the father blames her for errors of commission and omission.

The third message comes from the negative model, which is in use in medicine in particular, but in other service professions as well. This is the model that does not incorporate or respect individual differences, and that therefore labels any deviation from a narrowly defined ideal or norm as pathological. This model gives a message to women that the changes and disruptions they experience in pregnancy are deviant and dangerous. The struggles they perceive and respond to in the first months and years with their developing children are defined as pathological and "abnormal."

The extent to which these messages devalue women's attempts to define themselves as mothers is increased by the unclear goals and standards of child rearing in our society. The one exception that is clear is the standard of cognitive achievement as an outcome measure for mothering. It is surely unrewarding as a standard, for it does not rely on a feedback system, which is what mothering most essentially involves.

Clinical research with women as mothers provides us with observations for creating a nonpathological model for describing the developmental stages of becoming a mother. By *nonpathological model*, we mean a system derived from strengths and used to look for the positive aspects of a situation, as opposed to a system based on and used to identify potential pathology. We feel that this model is useful for understanding normal attachment and for finding more effective ways to cope with many of the situations faced by mothers today.

This developmental model begins preconceptually with the decision to become a mother. More and more, this decision is becoming a controlled and conscious act, rather than an "accident" as a result of some other goal. This phenomenon of planned parenting sets the stage for conscious, active involvement in the relationship with and responsibility toward the child. It has long been recognized that the mother–infant relationship starts during pregnancy.[3] The turmoil and anxiety of readjustment to the new role have often been viewed as tumultuous and even as pathological. In our work with pregnant women, as we interview them as their prospective pediatricians, we have come to view this disruptive process as functional. The mother-to-be is working through an important developmental stage: the uprooting of old attachments. That it occurs and that it appears to be so disruptive is a necessary first step in preparing for a new, important attachment. She must mobilize psychic energy to be available for organizing around the new infant, energy that is freed in such a coping system.

A major feature of this disruptive state is ambivalence. Preparation includes the mobilization of both positive and negative feelings. These are expressed in her feelings about herself as a mother, as she works out the clarity and the confidence with which she will approach the new role. This ambivalence will underlie all of her feelings toward the child. It will be reflected in her expectations, hopes, and fears for the child and in her relationship with her or him. The total symbiosis of pregnancy and the relative symbiosis of the first few postpartum months must gradually be replaced by an attached, loving relationship, but one that will allow for the autonomy and the individuality of both mother and child. The negative side of the ambivalence, therefore, plays a necessary role in allowing the mother to break the initial symbiosis and to allow the child to separate from her.

With delivery, the importance of preparation in pregnancy becomes clear.[4] Now the available energy is consolidated around the new, individual infant. A major step has occurred. The wide range of possibilities for individuality in the baby, to which a woman must remain open during pregnancy, is narrowed by the reality of the infant. The infant brings uniqueness in terms of his or her particular combination of behavioral, temperamental, and physical characteristics and finally provides a solid entity to the mother for attachment. The individuality can be met more effectively because of the amount of energy mobilized during pregnancy (because of the disruption of old ties and the ambivalence), which can now be focused on the real infant.

It is important to keep in mind that the development of attachment now becomes a two-way process. The mother learns about her infant and the time it takes to learn will be based on her previous child-care experiences and her needs and expectations from a child. The child is learning about the mother through a variety of rather impressive skills of discrimination, by virtue of which she or he will modify, but not completely change, her or his complex behavioral and temperamental repertoire. In recent years, much research has been focused on these skills and behaviors of the newborn. Some specific examples may be useful here.

At birth, the infant can fix on and follow visual stimuli, both animate and inanimate, and is alert to and turns to appropriate auditory stimuli.[5] Even an ability to discriminate ranges of pitch is demonstrable at birth, and the infant turns preferentially to higher-pitched, female voices.

Within a week, the infant selects by smell her or his own mother's breast pads, rather than another woman's.[6] By 4 weeks of age, the infant demonstrates a recognition of his or her mother's voice, by turning to it more frequently than to another woman's voice, and smiles and attends more to his or her mother's face.[7]

Sander et al. have studied the ways in which newborns use these powers of discrimination to adapt their own behavior.[8,9] Cassell and Cassell and Sander have reported on a study of normal newborns cared for by their own mothers for two weeks in a lying-in hospital in England. During the first 10 days of normal care by the mothers, he observed and recorded the infants' state changes, that is, the patterns of sleep, drowsy, awake, and crying cycles that the infants moved through during a 24-hour period. By the end of 10 days, these patterns were regular and predictable for each infant, and the regularity was related to the contacts, particularly in feeding, with the mother. On the morning of the 11th day, the mothers wore ski masks during the first feed. The infants' regular patterns of state changes were disrupted for the next four to six hours and only then slowly returned to normal.

Gould carried out a similar experiment, this time recording electroencephalograms (EEGs) (through which state changes can be observed even more accurately) on infants cared for by nurses in a hospital nursery for the first two weeks of life. He found that when an infant was fed every four hours by the same nurse, his or her EEG pattern of state changes became more predictable, mature, and regular. The maturation began to occur after only three or four feedings. When a new nurse fed the infant, the EEG pattern regressed and became less regular. The regularity returned gradually over the next two to three feedings with the same nurse.

These few examples point up the skill of the newborn in discriminating among caregivers and in using those discriminations for adaptations at all levels, even a level as basic as brain maturation. The studies have heightened our appreciation of the role of the infant in the development of attachment; these skills appear to be the building blocks.

Our understanding of the readiness of a woman to become attached to her infant at its birth is heightened by the work of Klaus et al.[10] They have studied the effects of close, immediate, private contact between a mother and her infant at birth as reflected in the later manifestations of attachment. They allowed the mothers 45 minutes of time with their nude infants immediately after delivery (rather than waiting the standard 12 hours for contact). In addition, they gave the mothers and infants four extra hours of contact per day in hospital. On followup (which ranged from one to five years), they found positive effects in several different areas, including the attachment behavior of the mothers at one year, and also in weight gain in the infants, the length of time breast feeding, the number of illnesses in the first year, and the language development in the children at 5 years of age.

At this time, we can only speculate on what aspect of the contact led to such profound, long-range effects. One possibility is the effect of the researchers' communicating to the mother that it was important for her and her infant to be together. Another possibility is that in the first few hours after delivery, newborns have a long period of quiet, awake alertness, during which time they may be particularly available to engaging in eye-to-eye contact with their mothers. They may, therefore, be more powerful elicitors of the mothers' positive feelings.

This is an area where similar mechanisms appear to be at work in the father–infant relationship. Fathers who have attended the delivery and who have had contact with their infants at birth describe a heightened sense of relatedness or belonging to the infant from the beginning. These more intense feelings of attachment, in fact, increase rather than decrease over time and are associated with a more complex, resilient, and rewarding relationship with the child.

All of this research leaves us with several clear messages. First, the infant is complex and competent in ways that are particularly suited to eliciting caretaking behavior and to learning about and adapting to the mother. Second, the infant demonstrates these capacities from birth, and, in fact, some may be particularly available in the few hours following delivery. Third, the work of pregnancy in mobilizing energy for attachment, as well as the physiological and psychological processes of labor and delivery, particularly prime the mother to become attached to the infant from birth.

The information has begun to lead us toward a more positive approach to examining and adapting delivery practices in this country, and it can provide us with guidelines for balancing the priorities necessary for a healthy outcome to pregnancy, both physical and emotional.

We can assume that modern obstetrical and neonatal practices, with their significant technical strides, will continue to monitor the important physical needs and to intervene when necessary. But within that context, we can now begin to construct a situation in which a woman can express her own choices and establish her autonomy as a prospective parent. This is not just a simple matter of giving her a feeling of power in the situation. Being autonomous in this uniquely female achievement is paramount to her own development as a woman. The autonomy is necessary to foster the positive side of her feelings of competence as a mother and to allow her to derive self-esteem from the role.

We can also begin to structure the early lying-in period to allow safe but earlier and more frequent contacts between mother and new-born. We emphasize the safe aspect of these contacts because of our observations in cultures living a more marginal, survival existence. These indicate the importance of early physical support for the mother, so that she can recover from delivery and so that her energy can be available not just to nurture the child but to attach herself to it and to foster its optimal emotional and cognitive development.

Understanding these individual elements in mother and infant at birth is the background for the next stage, that of understanding the interaction as it develops. The interaction incorporates these preg-nancy and perinatal processes, and in particular, the continuing clari-fication and expression of the woman's feelings toward herself and her child, as well as the continuing discriminatory powers of the infant. But the interaction has another characteristic: its reciprocity. By *rec-iprocity*, we mean that both partners negotiate through interaction for a fulfilling relationship with feedback that is based on each of their individual needs.

It is through reciprocity that mother and child form the essential attachment; but of equal importance to the formation of attachment is individualization and the growth of autonomy in each member. Rec-iprocity allows for individualization, which is necessary to ego devel-opment. And individualization, in turn, acts as a powerful energizer to the relationship.

We will describe some of the stages and processes in the devel-opment of the interaction, but first, we need to present the obvious but important framework within which they take place. The human newborn, as unique from other mammals, even from subhuman pri-mates, has a long period of motor dependency, during which close physical contact is essential for her or his survival. She or he is not autonomously mobile for at least six months, and only gradually after that. In the meantime, the infant must be tended and carried; this ensures close proximity with a caregiver. In contrast to the motor sphere, the human infant is the most precocious socially and affec-tively (e.g., social orientation skills at birth and social-affective com-munication through smiles, vocalizations, and facial expression are rich and effective by 1–2 months of age). This combination of prolonged motor dependency and precocious social development allows for the early and effective transmission of complex messages for acculturation, through attachment and identification to uniquely powerful individ-uation. In other words, human infancy seems designed to produce the complexity of human adulthood. We believe that the reciprocal interaction between mother and infant is the most important mediator of this process.

The first author's studies of early reciprocal interaction began with the observation that an infant's behavior and attention were completely different at as early as 3 weeks of age when the infant was interacting with its mother as opposed to another adult or with an object.[11] When an object was brought into the infant's visual field and then into "reach space," the infant would fix on it, her or his face would brighten, and attention would build rapidly to an intense visual exploration of the object. This period of intense, continuous attention ended abruptly with the infant's turning away, to stare neutrally at a distant object or, often, at nothing. After a brief period of "recuperation," the infant would then turn back to the object for another period of intense exploration. During the periods of attention, the infant's movements were jerky and pointing in the direction of the object. (These movements are now seen as the component precursors to reaching.)

With the mother, the pattern of attention was completely different. The long periods of attention achieved with her were actually composed of many shorter periods of attention and nonattention, which cycled in a smooth, rhythmical fashion at a rate of four times per minute. The infant would cycle with the mother, through attention and nonattention and from positive affect to neutral disengagement. The infant's body movements, too, were different. They were now softened and smooth and, in fact, cycled in a smooth approach–withdrawal pattern, in rhythm with the attentional cycle. This interaction was striking when there was reciprocity; the attentional cycles formed a smooth, homeostatic curve of involvement and rest for both partners, as they locked into an interaction with each other. The infant's cycle was matched to the mother's; she moved in with peak affective information while the infant was attending and withdrew or let up on the intensity of affect as the infant disengaged.

It is difficult to imagine a more appropriate system than this homeostatic, reciprocal interaction. The homeostatic attentional cycle is economical in allowing long periods of attention without exhausting the infant and, at the same time, facilitating the richest affective communication. It is superbly adaptive for balancing the infant's physiological demands and its psychological needs. It is a flexible system for addressing the infant's need for qualitatively different interactions with a few important caregivers.

Specifically, our studies with fathers and infants showed that by 3–4 weeks of age, infants were achieving interactions with their fathers that were qualitatively different from their interactions with their mothers, but with the same element of reciprocal affective control at work. [12] The infant not only passively discriminated caregivers at this age but actively engaged in a differentiated interaction. The father, with interactional goals different from the mother's had provided the infant with the opportunity for expressing and experiencing a variation on the reciprocal interactional theme.

We have now been able to characterize the amount of affective and cognitive information transmitted in such an interaction, as well as the degree of reciprocity achieved. [13] We have seen several patterns in "failing" interactions. Where the mother is too anxious or insensitive and overwhelms the infant by not recognizing or respecting the withdrawal part of the homeostatic curve, the infant remains almost entirely disengaged, although continuously monitoring her in peripheral vision.

When the pair cannot get into reciprocal homeostasis and when the affective and cognitive information is not cycled, the infant's attentional pattern begins to resemble that of a more expansive, unilateral model. We have also been able to discover in pairs in which the infant is afflicted and the physiological demands outstrip the psychological demands, that the baby and the mother cannot get into a reciprocal interaction at first, but that over time, they finally begin to learn about each other. The pair will "make it" when the mother can use even brief periods of attention available in the infant or can find other ways of establishing reciprocity.

What does such reciprocal interaction mean? Our cross-cultural work indicates that it is through early affective communication that a society transmits its affective values and patterns and molds them to the individual, and vice versa. Our studies of this early interaction in other cultures demonstrate that the reciprocal nature and the infant's skills in discriminating are present by the very early age of 3 weeks. We found, however, that the specific modalities and patterns through which the reciprocity and discrimination are manifest differ from culture to culture. The differences are related to factors ranging from the particular affective goals for an adult member of the culture to the level of nutrition available in the society.

For example, we have studied these reciprocal interactions among the Gusii tribe of Kenya, where there are taboos against, and avoidance of, intense affective expression, especially in face-to-face interactions among adults. [14] The Gusii mothers and their infants at 3 months of age engage in the same type of reciprocally controlled interaction, but with two important differences from the American sample. The Gusii infants maintained a positive affective state even though their mothers abruptly broke the homeostatic cycle; when the Gusii mothers sat still-faced in front of their infants (a condition that causes American infants of the same age to become withdrawn and to show increasing negative affect), the Gusii infants, after a brief attempt to elicit a response from their mothers, were able to maintain an even, positive affective state and to direct their attention elsewhere without becoming withdrawn.

It appeared to us that by 3 months of age, at least, the Gusii rules for social-affective interactions were at work and were being transmitted, as in the American sample.

In an elegant study by Chavez, improvements in the pregnant women's and their infants' nutritional states had a cascadelike effect in increasing the types of relationships that the infants were seen engaging in, in part by increasing the infants' own initiating role and by involving more caretakers, most particularly the father.[15]

Chavez's study and the nutritional affects we saw in our Gusii sample seem to indicate that under such stress as malnutrition, energy may be conserved by restriction in the area of this reciprocal interaction. But this restriction leaves the infant without the opportunity for rich and varied interactions, in which he or she is an active partner, and may, therefore, be one of the mediating factors in the detrimental effect of malnutrition on later functioning.

When the interaction fails completely in our culture, it means the potential for a disastrous situation, such as failure to thrive or child abuse.

But what is most relevant to this paper is what this reciprocal interaction means in most mother–infant pairs in our culture, those that are normal and healthy. In these situations, it is the basis of the mother–child relationship. For the infant, it is the setting in which his or her individuality will be recognized at its psychological-physiological interface. As a result, it is the setting in which the infant's affective development will be fueled, as well as its cognitive experiences elaborated.

For the mother, the feedback from a successful interaction, in which the pair are "making it," is an invaluable and constant reminder in securing her own positive feelings about her mothering capacities. The feedback information that through this mutual interaction she can nurture and support her infant provides the fuel for her actually to continue and grow with that role. In addition, a successful interaction means that the mother has recognized her infant's active role, as well as her own, in the infant's development. This recognition is essential for the healthy development of their relationship, bringing them from symbiosis to autonomy.

We, as pediatricians, see this reciprocal interaction at work in every pivotal developmental event in the first year of life. There are three such events in particular that are clearly defined and that act as markers for us of the successful negotiation of the relationship.

The first event occurs around the end of the second postpartum week. Pediatricians are aware of this time through the classical "two-week anxiety" phone call from every new mother and many experienced ones. Without an understanding of the developmental processes involved, the response to the call is either annoyance or blanket reassurance. Developmentally, in the third week, most mothers are at a complex psychological and physiological crossover point. They are aware of a nadir of energy, but they are not always aware that this means that physiological recovery is beginning its upswing. They are at a peak realization of the complexity of their task, but also just at the point of being able to recognize the positive individual aspects of the baby, and the interaction these make possible. The gradual relinquishment of fantasy for reality, as a basis for personifying and individualizing the infant, is beginning.

Instead of giving blanket reassurance about the future, the actual and immediate positive aspects of these psychological and physiological curves can be addressed by a supportive caregiver. Most women are able to respond when they see the limits of their responsibility for themselves and get the feedback confirming their right to enjoy the interaction. Then, they can overcome the energy drain and the anxiety generated by the earlier and continuing ambivalence about their new, demanding role.

Here is a place where the father's separate and unique interaction and relationship with the child, which is just beginning to take shape, is enormously helpful. The existence of such a separate relationship demonstrates to the mother (1) that the infant is a separate individual, not just responding to and dependent on her; and (2) that another caregiver (or several others, e.g., siblings or extended-family members) can respond to some of the infant's needs so that the mother is not solely responsible for covering the entire spectrum of possible interactions and relationships. This effect of the father's active involvement with the infant is first brought to bear as early as this 3- to 4-week crisis time and can be a continuing source of both enrichment and dilution of the mother–infant interaction throughout infancy and early childhood.

Another pivotal event occurs around 3–4 months of age. At this stage, the infant begins to act voluntarily, separately from the mother. One of the most common manifestations is the interruption of a feeding, the baby turning away from the mother and investing its interest elsewhere. The infant actively chooses to direct its attention away from the mother and refuses to be drawn back.

When the relationship is going well prior to this, it can provide support for the positive feelings, so that the other side of the reciprocity coin can be expressed: the acceptance of the infant's autonomy. In this positive relationship, the mother's ambivalence comes to the surface. The mother must recognize it, and she can then begin the necessary separation. In the process, she further conquers her ambivalence. If, on the other hand, the interaction is not going well, the ambivalence generates anxiety. The mother may fix on the infant's developing autonomy as a symptom of their failure in the reciprocity. The feeding situation becomes a battleground. Or the autonomy struggle may continue in other spheres, such as sleep. The mother may cling to the symbiosis in this area and not allow the infant to begin to deal autonomously with her or his own sleep–wake cycles. When the infant cries, she may not be able to allow the infant to make full use of her or his capacity to deal with getting back to sleep, and she may set up too dependent a relationship at night.

Intervention at this point may consist in pointing out the infant's needs and capacities for autonomy, but always within the context of recognizing with the mother what this may mean for her.

A third stage occurs around 8 or 9 months of age with the concurrent emergence of three themes: (1) the clear attachment of the infant to mother (with a definite expression of preference for her and protest at separation from her); (2) the classical stranger anxiety; and (3) active autonomy, whereby the infant is now not only insistent on controlling her or his attention but also on actually doing for herself or himself. The emergence of these three phenomena is related to a development in the cognitive sphere, where a clearer understanding of the permanence of objects and persons and a clear differentiation of self from others are occurring.

This is a particularly difficult time because of the contradictory messages from the child: insistence on the mother's presence and insistence on active autonomy. It seems that this is a point at which the mother's negotiation of her independence from her own past plays a role. If she has not completed that struggle herself, as a mother, or has been unsuccessful, watching her own child's struggle, and all of the ambivalence in it, is a threat instead of a tolerable and exciting process.

These are only three examples of the crucial developmental issues in the early mother–child relationship. Autonomy must be achieved by both mother and child, along with attachment; both are made possible by the reciprocal interaction.

We find this framework for understanding both sides of attachment–separation invaluable in our work as pediatricians, and we believe that it can be applied in programs affecting mothers and infants and their families.

The other supports available for young mothers include infant stimulation and day care or nurseries. The use of the positive developmental model (based on an understanding of the important reciprocal interaction) may help stimulation programs to redirect their efforts toward supporting the mother–infant relationship rather than just the infant's cognitive or motor skills. This framework may also enable day-care workers to capitalize on their potential for being a cohesive rather than a divisive influence on young families. The competition that inevitably develops between adults who care for young children (and that is understandable because it reflects the extent of their commitment to the children) may be more effectively dealt with in both these situations. It certainly helps us as part of a medical support system to participate in the developing mother–infant relationship and to support it more fully, both when it is evolving optimally and when it appears to be stressed. The model provides a powerful demonstration of how rewarding and how difficult is the developmental step of becoming a mother.

References

1. Deutsch H: *The psychology of women: Motherhood.* Vol. 2. New York, Grune & Stratton, 1945.
2. Bronfenbrenner U: The origins of alienations, *Scientific American* 231:53–62, 1974.
3. Bibring G, Dwyer TF, Huntington DS: A study of psychological processes in pregnancy and of the earliest mother child relationship, *Psychoanalytic Study of the Child* 16:9–24, 1961.
4. Brazelton TB: The early mother–infant adjustment, *Pediatrics* 32:931–938, 1963.
5. Brazelton TB: *Neonatal Behavioral Assessment Scale,* Clinics in Developmental Medicine, #50. London, Spastics International Medical Publications; Philadelphia, Lippincott, 1973.
6. MacFarlane JA: Olfaction in the development of social preferences in the human neonate. *Parent infant interaction,* CIBA Foundation Symposium #33. Amsterdam, Associated Scientific Publishers, 1975.
7. Wolff PH: Observations on the early development of smiling. In *Determinants of infant behavior.* Edited by Foss BM. New York, Wiley, 1963.
8. Cassel T, Sander L: *Neonatal recognition processes and attachment: The masking experiment.* Paper presented at Biennial Meeting of the Society for Research in Child Development, August 1975.
9. Sander L, Chappel P, Gould J, Snyder P: *An investigation of change in the infant caretaker system over the first week of life.* Paper presented at the Biennial Meeting of the Society for Research in Child Development, April 1975.
10. Klaus MH, Jerauld R, Kreger NC: Maternal attachment: Importance of the first postpartum days, *New England Journal of Medicine* 286:460–463, 1972.

11. Brazelton TB: Origins of reciprocity. In *The effect of the infant on its caregiver.* Edited by Lewis M, Rosenblum L. New York, Wiley, 1973.
12. Yogman MW, Dixon S, Tronick E, Brazelton TB: *The goals and structure of face-to-face interaction between infants and fathers.* Paper presented at the Meeting of the Society for Research in Child Development, New Orleans, March 1977.
13. Brazelton TB, Tronick E, Adamson L, Als H, Wise S: Early mother–infant reciprocity. *Parent Infant Interaction,* CIBA Foundation Symposium #33. Amsterdam, Elsevier/Excerpta Medica/North Holland, 1975. pp 137–154
14. Keefer C, Dixon S, Tronick E, Brazelton TB: *The structure of infant–adult social reciprocity: A cross-cultural study of face-to-face interaction: Gusii infants and mothers.* Paper presented at the Meeting of the Society for Research in Child Development, New Orleans, March 1977.
15. Chavez A, Martinez C, Yashine T: *Nutrition, mother–child relations and behavioral development in the young child from a rural community.* Unpublished manuscript of Instituto Nacional de Nutricion, Mexico City, 1973.

Chapter 6

To Marry or Not to Marry

CAROL NADELSON AND MALKAH NOTMAN

Although the number of people who choose to remain single has increased over the past decade, about 95% of contemporary Americans are still expected to marry at some time in their lives.[1] This statistic represents a slight *increase* over the early part of the century. Despite the fact that an increasing proportion of the under-30 group has never married, the proportion of the population reaching their 40s without marrying is at an all-time low. This trend may signal postponement, but it may also mean that a larger proportion of younger people will never marry, a phenomenon that can have major societal implications.

In the past, few women chose not to marry, because remaining unmarried carried with it a strong social stigma, as well as economic problems. An unmarried woman was seen as unattractive, unworthy, and unwanted. Women also felt this way about themselves. They experienced considerable pressure to marry, in order to feel "chosen." The decision they made was not whether to marry, but whom to marry, and perhaps when.

In the early 1950s, when Kuhn studied a group of men and women who had not married, the reasons given for remaining unmarried were expressed in negative terms.[2] These included hostility toward marriage or toward members of the opposite sex, lack of interest in heterosexual partners, emotional involvement with parents, poor health, feelings of physical unattractiveness, unwillingness to assume responsibility, inability to find one's "true love," a sense of social inadequacy, perception of marriage as a threat to career goals, economic

---

CAROL NADELSON, M.D., AND MALKAH NOTMAN, M.D. • Department of Psychiatry, Tufts University School of Medicine–New England Medical Center Hospital, Boston, Massachusetts.

problems, and geographic, educational, or occupational isolation, which limited the chances of meeting an eligible mate.

A recent study by Stein cited more positive reasons for choosing to remain single.[3] Both men and women spoke of increased freedom and enjoyment of life, opportunities to meet people and develop friendships, economic independence, and more and better social experience and opportunities for personal development. Adams suggested that in order for a woman's choice to remain single to be a successful adaptation, she must be economically independent, be socially and psychologically autonomous, and have a clear preference for being single.[4]

An indication of the magnitude of the attitudinal change regarding marriage can be seen in studies done at different times. A 1962 study of unmarried college students revealed that only 2% of them had little or no interest in future marriage.[5] A decade later, 40% of senior women said they did not know whether they would marry. Further, 39% of seniors felt that traditional marriage was becoming obsolete. Bird believes that changes in sexual mores and sex roles have contributed to this attitude change. She stated that men no longer marry to have sexual partners and women no longer marry for financial support.[6] Although it was not possible to accurately predict the future behavior of those students who stated that they were not interested in marriage, the difference in stated attitudes and expectations from 1962 to 1972 was striking.

There have been few studies that have examined, in depth, the reasons for remaining single. It is clear that the picture is a complex one and that the determinants are multiple, even for a given person. In addition to socioeconomic and educational factors, homosexuality, childhood experience of parents' marital unhappiness or divorce and the absence of the desire for children are important. Changing societal and sexual attitudes have made it possible for both men and women to fulfill their needs for intimate relationships without marriage and to engage in a greater range of activities as single people than was possible in the past.

There are also important unconscious reasons for not marrying, including anxieties about commitment, difficulties in sustaining relationships, and feelings about marriage deriving from early experiences with one's parents. While these have probably always existed, current social patterns and changes in expectations permit their expression in life choices to a greater extent.

Several studies have shown that the frequency of the intention not to marry or the postponement of the desired time for marriage in-

creases with more education.[7,8,9,10] An examination of the characteristics of working single women indicates a bimodal distribution: one
age group is young and uneducated, and the other group is older and
better educated. Many of those in the younger group are likely to marry
at some later time, whereas many of the more educated, older group
are likely to meet Adams's criteria for successful adaptation to remaining single and to decide not to marry.[11,12] For these women, other
goals and values replace traditional expectations.

Unforeseen circumstances may also dictate the choice to remain
unmarried. Many women have had to care for elderly parents or for
siblings; others have life experiences, such as the loss of a fiancé or
other tragedies, which make marriage a less important or available
option for them. Some couples do not marry because of economic considerations; for example, they may lose tax or social security benefits
if they do marry.

In addition to those women who remain single because they have
never married, there are those who are widowed or divorced. It is
highly likely that at some point in her adult life, every woman will be
single for a time because of the current high divorce rate and the differential longevity of men and women. Although many of the concerns
of all single women are similar, this chapter focuses on those women
who choose to remain single.

LIFE EXPERIENCES FOR THE SINGLE WOMAN

While there are few studies of individuals who have chosen to
remain single, there do appear to be differences between the life experiences of single men and single women. Single women report greater
freedom and autonomy than married women, but they often find
themselves frustrated in their attempts at intimacy and in relationships with men. They may also feel socially isolated and lonely. Minority status brings with it confusion on the part of others with regard
to their roles, as well as confusion about how to relate to a "single"
woman. Friendships become an important source of support and
sustenance. Many single women live together or with their parents or
families for emotional or economic support.[13]

Remaining single seems to some women to provide advantages
for personal and professional development. It offers freedom from conflicts and the inevitable day-to-day negotiations with a spouse, as well
as an opportunity for solitude, self-reflection, and autonomous decision-making. The single woman may find enormous gratification in
her self-sufficiency, and this choice may be both adaptive and person-

ally rewarding. The advantages and the disadvantages coexist, and each woman must weigh these. For some, the positive aspects of remaining single emerge after an unhappy experience with marriage. For others, they support a reluctance to marry perhaps until a later life phase.

LIVING ALONE OR TOGETHER WITHOUT MARRIAGE

Living alone and living together without marriage have become increasingly acceptable options either for a short while or as a lifestyle, although there are indications that most single people do say they eventually want to marry. The proportion of young single people, particularly women, who establish their own households increased from 21% of 25- to 34-year-olds in 1970 to 29% of this age group in 1975. Many of these people, however, were not spending all their time alone. The number of couples who were making the decision to live together without marrying increased by 800% during the 1960s.[11]

The reasons given for this choice are complex. Some couples disapprove of marriage as an institution, others cite the desire to establish and test the viability of a relationship before making a permanent commitment. Loneliness, disillusionment with the superficiality of the "dating game," and the search for intimacy combined with a reluctance to make a permanent commitment are also important reasons for living together.

For some couples, this arrangement works well and is an impetus to further development and maturation. For others, it becomes confusing and is a potential source of anxiety and conflict. A premature decision to live together by young people who have not explored other relationships may actually interfere with personal maturation and the development of sexual identity, although it may appear that the couple has achieved just these things by making the decision to live together. Anxiety often occurs when the nature of the relationship is not explicit, leaving many fantasied expectations and increasing the possibility of disappointment.

There are no consistent patterns of interaction in these couples. Their relationships differ with regard to lifestyles and the contracts between the partners. Some couples feel committed to each other and see their relationship as similar to marriage; others are transiently attached or even merely sharing the convenience of housing or cooking.

For some young people, the nonmarital living situation is a way of working out the patterns of interaction before they can marry. Their concept of marriage includes a high degree of intimacy and mutual sharing, which they expect can evolve before they make the decision to marry. It is important to understand these decisions in relation to the particular developmental phase of a given individual or couple.

DEVELOPMENTAL CONSIDERATIONS

The young adult years (18–21) are generally considered the time of separation from the family of origin and of preparation for major adult roles. These include the stabilization of gender identity, the choice of occupational role, the development of intimate relationships, and the deepening of commitment to one's own interests and values.[14,15]

Young men and women presumably face similar developmental tasks; however, the pressure of making a commitment to an occupational choice has been higher for men, historically. Although there are indications that this is changing, marriage has been perceived as women's central adult role, and their other activities have been regarded as subordinate to and contingent on future family functions.[16,17] Work and career choices have been thought of as temporary. Most women learned early in their lives that the choice of a husband, not a career or a job, was the most important determinant of their future.[18] Indeed, until the census of 1980, a woman's socioeconomic status has been decided in relation to that of her father or her husband. Therefore, in the early adult phases of development, young women have maintained some tentativeness in the evolution of their personal identity, and they have waited until marriage defined the context of their lives.[15,19,20] Since a clear definition of a woman's needs, values, goals, satisfactions, and activities may limit her choices in potential mate selection, maintenance of flexibility and openness is more adaptive for increasing marital options. However, it may compromise the development of career goals as well as inhibit the differentiation of the individual.[18] This pattern of suspending commitment is more an issue for women than for men, since men have usually expected women to adapt to their careers and lifestyles.

Gilligan noted that for men, "identity" precedes "intimacy" and "generativity," in the Eriksonian model of the optimal cycle of human development. For women, however, these tasks seem to be joined, and intimacy accompanies identity.[21] Women have defined themselves and become identified in the world through their relationships with others. Thus, the stages of ego development through the life cycle appear to differ for men and women. Women also appear to be more dependent on others for support, approval, and direction than men.[17,22] For women, the young adult period has been conceptualized as a transitional period from dependence on their parents to dependence on their spouse.[17]

From a developmental perspective, men and women who marry early, before they have settled their concerns about identity and independence, may find their choices inappropriate later. Some individuals are prepared to cope with the tasks of marriage at an early age; others may still be burdened by excessive dependency needs, unrealistic expectations of their partners, or unresolved psychological issues, which make the commitment to an intimate relationship difficult or premature. While some who enter marriage when they are less mature can grow within it, others who either cannot cope with the stress or cannot resolve past conflicts or trauma are vulnerable to disturbance.

WHY MARRY?

In a discussion of the reasons not to marry, one must also consider the reasons for choosing marriage. As we have indicated, the reasons for choosing marriage are complex. For the individual, marriage represents a way of fulfilling personal desires for happiness, security and companionship, social role expectations, economic security, and confirmation of being worthwhile and "chosen." These reasons have been particularly compelling for women, although the married state carries its problems. In our culture, the decision to marry is also frequently based on romantic expectations of what marriage and the marital partner will be like, rather than on more practical considerations.

Many of the psychological theories that have been offered to account for mate selection are variants of exchange theory. They propose a marriage market analogous to the economic market in which goods and services are exchanged.[23,24,25,26,27] The implication is that the greater the desirability of the characteristics a person has to offer to the opposite sex, the "more" he or she will obtain in a spouse. There is an implicit assumption of certain "universal" values and attitudes, for example, that most women place a high emphasis on status-conferring ability in seeking husbands, and that men emphasize physical attractiveness in seeking wives. These views, of course, neglect the importance of personal values and psychological variables in making a deliberate choice to marry or not to marry. The marketplace analogy supports the view that if one is not "chosen," it is because of insufficient assets, rather than because there are positive, or even neurotic, reasons for the choice not to marry.

The desire to have children continues to be an important reason for marriage for most women. Although there are increasing numbers of single mothers, this pattern is not usually a deliberate choice, except for a small minority of women who bear or adopt children because the desire for motherhood overrides their desire for marriage, or they do not feel that they will marry. This latter group continues to be small and has not been well studied.

Childless marriage is, of course, possible. For the first time in human history, the choice to be childless without sacrificing sexuality is possible for large numbers of people because of the availability of effective contraceptives and abortion. The consequences of this change are not yet clear. However, without children, one of the usual reasons for marriage is eliminated. Couples often do not marry until they want a child or the woman becomes pregnant. Veevers has reported that about 5% of all married couples voluntarily forgo parenthood. For approximately one-third of childless couples, the decision not to have children is made before marriage.[28]

Another important consideration in the decision to marry involves family and friends' expectations and pressures. Parents often see the failure of their offspring to marry as a measure of their own failure in the parental role. They may be concerned, particularly when they have a single daughter, that she will be alone and uncared for. They also feel deprived of grandparenthood. Friends and acquaintances are often concerned because the single person may be viewed as a "threat" to the relationship and the stability of married people.[29]

There are also pressures from the workplace. There are reports of active discrimination against single people. For example, 80% of the companies reporting in Jacoby's 1974 survey asserted that while marriage was not essential to upward mobility, the majority of executives and junior management were married.[30] Over 60% felt that single executives tend to make snap judgments, and 25% believed that single people are less stable than married people.

Just as the desire to remain single has unconscious determinants and may derive from conflict and anxiety about closeness, intimacy, or sharing, the desire to marry also derives, in part, from unconscious issues. These include strong needs for dependency, failure to separate or to develop a secure independent indentity, intolerable fear of isolation or loneliness, and more positively, identification with parents and needs for autonomy. Marriage itself is not indicative of psychological health or maturity.

The Impact of Marriage on Women

Demographic data indicate that the married state appears to be associated with more stress for women than for men. Married women seek help for physical and emotional problems more often than married men or single women.[31,32,33,34,35] There have been several reasons offered for this disparity:[13]

1. The woman who marries modifies her life more than her husband does and risks more loss of autonomy. Although this is changing, and there are an increasing number of couples who work out alternative shared lifestyles, nontraditional patterns are by no means problem-free, nor do they necessarily change some of the pressures of family life.

2. For women who marry and become housewives, there is a tendency toward lack of role differentiation. The housewife role is an ascribed rather than an achieved role, and it is expected that women perform well in it without opportunity for diversification. Women feel that they must succeed in it, but because the standards for being a successful homemaker are vague, any experience perceived as failure can lead to symptoms, including low self-esteem and depression. The housewife role can also be isolating, allowing few opportunities for adult interchange and support, particularly when children are small.

3. A loss of status may occur for a woman who has had an active career and then gives it up to marry. She often finds her role as housewife and mother devalued, although superficial attention is paid to its importance. While fewer women without children now give up work, many women alter their career or work patterns and take positions with more flexibility and fewer time demands in order to spend more time at home or to be available to their husbands to entertain or to meet other demands.

From her data on marital satisfactions, as well as patterns of illness, Bernard has concluded that marriage is more beneficial to men than to women.[17] However, Glenn concluded that while married women exceed men in the stress that they experience, they also derive more satisfaction from marriage.[36] The apparent contradictions are based on which aspects of marriage are examined. Although marriage is associated with certain indications of stress in women, singleness is also experienced as stressful in different ways.

CONCLUSION

It is too early to know which direction women will take, and current trends may be transient. However, the changing role of women in society and the emergence of the possibility of reproductive control, two clearly related phenomena, have enabled women, for the first time in history, to have greater choice in the direction of their lives. This change has also had an impact on men's roles, and it is hoped that it will provide both men and women the freedom to choose, in ways suitable to each, rather than yielding to expectations that do not take account of individual needs or differences.

References

1. Glick P: Demographer looks at American families, *Journal of Marriage and the Family* 37:15–26, 1975.
2. Kuhn M: How mates are sorted, in *Family, marriage and parenthood.* Edited by Becker H, Hill R. Boston, Heath, 1955.
3. Stein P: *Single in America.* Englewood Cliffs, N. J., Prentice-Hall, 1976.
4. Adams M: The single women in today's society, *American Journal of Orthopsychiatry* 41:776–786, 1971.
5. Bell R: *Marriage and family interaction.* Homewood, Ill., Dorsey, 1971.
6. Bird C: The case against marriage, in *The future of the family.* Edited by Howe, L. K. New York, Simon & Schuster, 1972.
7. Taylor T, Glenn ND: The utility of education and attractiveness for female status attainment through marriage, *American Sociologic Review* 41:484–498, 1976.
8. Glenn ND, Ross AA, Tully JC: Patterns of intergenerational mobility of females through marriage, *American Sociologic Review* 39:683–699, 1974.
9. Davis J: *Great aspirations.* Chicago, Aldine Press, 1964.
10. Ginzberg E: *Lifestyles of educated women.* New York, Columbia University Press, 1966.
11. U.S. Bureau of the Census: *Current Population Reports. Marital Status and Living Arrangements.* U. S. Government Printing Office, *March 1976.*
12. Donelson E, Gullahorn J: *Women: A psychological perspective.* New York, Wiley, 1977.
13. Frieze I, Parsons J, Johnson P, Ruble D, Zellman G: *Women and sex roles.* New York, Norton, 1978.
14. White R: *Lives in progress: A study of the natural growth of personality,* (2nd ed.). New York, Holt, Reinhard & Winston, 1966.
15. Erikson E: *Identity: Youth and crisis.* New York, Norton, 1968.
16. Kuhlen R, Johnson G: Changes in goals with adults' increasing age, *Journal of Consulting Psychology* 16 (1):1–4, 1952.
17. Bernard J: *Women, wives and mothers: Values and options.* Chicago, Aldine, 1975.
18. Angrist S, Almquist E: *Careers and contingencies: How college women juggle with gender.* New York, Dunellen, 1975.
19. Lowenthal M, Thurnher N, Chiriboga D: *Four stages of life: A comparative study of women and men facing transitions.* San Francisco, Jossey-Bass, 1975.
20. Douvan E, Adelson J: *The adolescent experience.* New York, Wiley, 1966.
21. Gilligan C: Woman's place in man's life cycle, *Harvard Educational Review* 49 (4):431–446, 1979.
22. Mischel W: A social learning view of sex differences and behavior, in *The development of sex differences.* Edited by Maccoby E. Stanford, Calif., Stanford University Press, 1966.
23. Waller W: *The family: A dynamic interpretation.* New York, Dryden Press, 1938.
24. Goode W: Family and mobility, in *Class, Status and Power* (2nd ed.). Edited by Bendix R, Lipset S. New York, New York Free Press, pp. 582–601, 1966.
25. Edwards J: Familial behavior as social exchange. *Journal of Marriage and the Family* 31:518–526, 1969.
26. Elder G: Appearance and education in marriage and mobility, *American Sociological Review* 43:510–533, 1969.

27. Murstein B: Stimulus-value-role: A theory of marital choice, *Journal of marriage and the Family* 32:465–482, 1970.
28. Veevers J: Voluntary childlessness: A review of issues and evidence, *Marriage and Family Review* 2 (2):1–26, 1979.
29. Duberman L: *Marriage and its alternatives*. New York, Praeger, 1974.
30. Jacoby S: 49-Million singles can't be all right, *The New York Times Magazine*, February 17, 1974.
31. Williams J: *Psychology of women: Selected readings*. New York, Norton, 1979.
32. Williams J: *Psychology of women*. New York, Norton, 1977.
33. Bernard J: *The future of marriage*. New York, Bantam, 1973.
34. Nadelson C, Notman M: The woman patient, in *The woman patient: Medical and psychological interfaces*. Vol. 1. Edited Notman M, Nadelson C. New York, Plenum Press, pp. 1–7, 1978.
35. Giele J: Changing sex roles and the future of marriage, in *Contemporary marriage: Structure, dynamics and therapy*. Edited by Grunebaum H, Christ J. Boston, Little, Brown, pp. 69–87, 1976.
36. Glenn ND: The contribution of marriage to the psychological well-being of males and females, *Journal of Marriage and the Family* 37:594–601, 1975.

Chapter 7

Maternal Work and Children

MALKAH NOTMAN AND CAROL NADELSON

Family patterns have changed considerably in the past 20 years. The increase in divorce, single-parent families, reconstituted families, and fathers receiving custody of children, as well as the enormous increase of women in the labor force, has made the conventionally structured family into a minority. In fact, in the past decade, families headed by women have grown in number 10 times as rapidly as two-parent families.[1] Many questions have arisen about the effects of these changes on families, and particularly on children.

At this time, only 6% of American families fit the traditional model of two parents, with the husband as the sole breadwinner and the wife at home caring for the children.[1,2] The "traditional" pattern itself, with a full-time mother who has no other occupation and remains in the house, has existed for a relatively short period of time. It evolved historically as a result of industrialization and the decline of the agricultural economy, which removed the site of industrial "work" from the home and thus separated the care of children from the paid employment. Furthermore, for women to spend this time solely in child care and housework when families are small demands relative affluence. In the past, women always filled many roles and shared the burden of work with their husbands in order to sustain their families. However, the work was most often at home and usually not for wages.

The number of women in the work force has increased enormously; it has grown by 60% in the past decade alone. Currently, more than one-half of all women 16 years or older are working outside the home or actively seeking employment. Of these women, 40% have

MALKAH NOTMAN, M.D. AND CAROL NADELSON, M.D. • Department of Psychiatry, Tufts University School of Medicine–New England Medical Center Hospital, Boston, Massachusetts.

children under 18 years of age, and 30% of children under 6 have working mothers.[1,2] Although the exact figures change with each year, the trend appears constant. Currently, most working women are married, are living with their husbands, and have school-age children. However, a large number, constituting more than 15 million, are single, separated, widowed, or divorced, and a large proportion of this group also has young children.

Responses to the changing role of women, including the increased number of women working, have ranged from complex attempts to understand the social changes and their consequences to simplistic, critical views, connecting the increase in time that women spend out of the home with divorce, teenage pregnancy, delinquency, violence, homosexuality, and other social "ills." Such positions fail to consider the multiple determinants of these changed social behaviors and the reciprocal relationships among them. Economic pressures have also constituted major reasons for women to work, and these have increased in the face of mounting inflation.

Concern about the welfare of children of working mothers is very legitimate, but it has been difficult to evaluate accurately. Child-care arrangements have varied enormously and often have not been considered in assessments of the effects of working mothers. This chapter focuses on the implications of the increased number of working mothers for children and families.

ATTITUDES TOWARD WORK AND CAREERS

Paralleling actual societal developments, there have been dramatic changes in the attitudes of young people about careers. Lozoff compared college students in 1965 and 1971 and found striking differences in attitudes between the earlier and later groups in the number of children that the students reported they wanted. In 1965, 2/3 of them wanted three or more children; in 1971, 1/6 wanted that number, and 1/10 wanted no children at all. Of the women students in 1967, 50% stated that having a career was important in addition to being a wife and mother. By 1971, this figure had risen to 81%.[3] Furthermore, in 1977, 91% of male students expressed interest in having a wife with a career, and 60% of both male and female students thought that fathers and mothers should spend equal time with children.[4] Although the pressures of the real situations that are encountered later tend to create differences between attitudes and behavior, these attitudinal changes do seem to be reflected in the work orientation and expectations of many people after college.

In 1971, Rapoport and Rapoport suggested that dual-career families would increase as more women worked, and that this change would require more arrangements for child care, further revisions in sex-role attitudes, and reconsiderations of the patterns of organization of productive work and family life.[5] In their subsequent volume, Rapoport and Rapoport pointed out that while the dual-career pattern is being chosen by more people, many aspects of the lifestyle of these couples still derive from the single-career pattern of interaction, decision making, and assumption of responsibility. Thus, the strains and pressures of dual careers have not changed.[6] These authors hypothesized that this lack of change was due to the inflexibility of social systems in adapting to potential changes, as well as to the internal resistance to change within individuals themselves, so that couples continued to do things in old ways even though these might be less effective in coping with new realities.

THE WORKING AND NONWORKING WOMAN

Most women work out of economic necessity. In spite of many gains in the careers open to women, most remain in low-status jobs with limited personal goals.[7] Moreover, they add their jobs to their traditional roster of home and family activities and often think of their work as an extension of their nurturant maternal and providing role. Few see it as an independent activity about which they may have some choice and from which they may expect personal gratification and the fulfillment of personal goals.[8] Women who work and have families often experience role strain as a result of the proliferation of their responsibilities.[9]

Any realistic assessment of the impact of the mother's work on her family's life or on her children must take a longitudinal perspective. Thus, childbearing and child rearing occupy only a relative small number of years, and a woman is often not prepared for a major part of her later life if she prepared herself primarily to be a mother and a caretaker of small children. In 1972, Rossi estimated that the average woman married at age 22, had two children two years apart, and died at 74, nine years after the husband's death at age 67. She thus had 56 years of adulthood starting from age 18:[10]

1. 23% of this period, or 13 years, was without a husband.
2. 41%, or 23 years, was with a husband but not with children under 18.
3. 36%, or 20 years, was with a husband and with children under 18.

Although increased life expectancy has changed the ways in which one needs to prepare for the future, many attitudes and values have persisted. Even if we assume that parenting is full time up to school age, or until the child is 6 years old, and that there are two children spaced two years apart, then only 12% of the period of caring for children (or 7 years) is spent on the full-time mothering of preschool children. While those specific figures also continue to change, it is clear that even the nonworking woman in contemporary society will spend almost two times as many years with neither husband nor dependent children as she does in carrying the responsibility for preschool children.

Rossi offered additional data about the amount of time a full-time mother spends on mothering. She calculated the actual time that middle-class housewives with young children spend on various activities. Her findings indicate that less than two hours per day are spent in direct mother–child interactions. The rest of the time is devoted to marketing, driving, errands, and household maintenance. Much of this time does indeed provide a background contact with the children, but the distracted or preoccupied mother is interacting in a very different way than the mother who is directly attending to her children.[10] Another interesting finding, from a study of specific work tasks after the increased availability of labor-saving devices, is that more time is spent on housework than in the past, presumably because women have become more exacting in their demands and expectations as a response to media influences and advertising, and they have more possessions to care for.[11]

Concern about changes in families must separate myths from the actual components of life for adult women. It is also important to consider the roles of men, with the possibilities for their sharing in the care of the children. The rising divorce rate raises another issue; many women will be alone for an even longer time than was true in the past. Many of them will need to support themselves, and often their children. Some of them will share custody of the children with the fathers or give up custody and face unexpected changes in mothering pattern and lifestyle.

INTEGRATION OF WORK AND FAMILIES

A consideration of the solutions to the work–career family dilemma in current society must therefore involve an assessment of the roles of all family members, including the husband's orientation to his family and his career, as well as the character of the work of both husband and wife. The assumption underlying the organization of the workplace has been that every man can or will spend a major portion of his energy and time on his work, but that women will not, and that they are therefore available for full-time attention to small children. Clearly, this assumption does not fit with prevailing realities, since most women are also working.

Women who work, however, still have a considerably greater feeling of responsibility for reconciling family and work demands than men have. This is heightened by the current reemphasis of the importance of early mother–infant relationships for the healthy development of children. Thus, mothers who work often feel guilty.

Even prior to the increase in the numbers of working women, there were indications that men valued the rewards of their family involvements more than was generally assumed, but little attention was paid to specific aspects of the role of husbands and fathers with regard to family integration until relatively recently.[5,6,12,13,14] The wife's career has hitherto been very dependent on the husband's adaptation and style, and it has been his decisions that have set the conditions for many aspects of family life.[15,16] Bailyn stated that the

> husband's mode of integrating family and work in his own life is crucial for success of any attempt of his wife to include a career in her life. . . . there is evidence that identifying the conditions under which men find it possible to give primary emphasis to their families while at the same time functioning satisfactorily in their own careers may be even more relevant to the problem of careers for married women than the continued emphasis on the difficulties women face in integrating family and work.[26]

IMPACT OF WORKING MOTHERS ON YOUNG CHILDREN

Concern and conflict about the care of their children are a prominent feature in the lives of mothers who work. If the children develop physical or emotional problems, the mothers are usually quick to be blamed and also blame themselves, although the actual causes of the problems may not be at all clear.[17] The working woman still often believes that her work is not in the best interest of her family. She may, in fact, overcompensate by asking for less help from other family members than the woman who is at home.[18]

The actual effects of maternal employment on children and families have been difficult to assess. The impact of maternal separation has been confused with data about maternal deprivation. Thus, it is often difficult to delineate the impact of each of these factors. The assumption has been made that separation is the same as deprivation, without adequately exploring the context and the degree of separation or deprivation and the available substitute care.

A growing body of data supports the idea that there are benefits for mother, children, and families when the mother works, even if it is out of necessity rather than desire. [19,20,21,22,23]

Many authors have emphasized the necessity of considering multiple variables in the context if we are to understand these issues, since to consider the effect of maternal employment alone is simplistic and thus limited in its applicability. [23,24,25] Obviously, the amount of time the mother is away; the quality of the family life; the presence of another parent, siblings, or other important people; and the developmental stage of the child–all are important in understanding the impact of the mother's working. So is the character of the work, the pleasure or burden it creates, and the flexibility or rigidity of the arrangements.

The literature on maternal-child attachment has brought new information and insights in the past years that have major implications for working mothers. Bowlby described the attachment that infants form with one primary caretaking person. [26] In their report on the effects of close contact between a mother and infant at birth and in the immediate postpartum period, Klaus and Kennell found that on follow-up, from one to five years, positive effects could be observed in a number of areas. [27] They demonstrated greater attachment behavior, greater infant weight gain, and fewer illnesses in the first year. There was greater language development at age 5 in those children who had had close contact as infants. These data would lead us to conclude that it may be detrimental for mothers to be separated from their very young infants for any reason, including work. There is, however, possibly contradictory evidence that indicates that the infant can form multiple attachments and that the strength of these attachments depends on the amount of attention it receives from its caretakers. [21,28,29] Thus, we can hypothesize that an infant whose mother was working, and who was therefore separated from her, could form additional attachments and benefit from these if they were consistent. In his review of the literature in this area, Rutter emphasized the quality of mothering as the critical variable. [28] He argued that the term *maternal deprivation* covers a range of responses and experiences not solely related to the absence of the mother. Schaeffer and Emerson have reported that the infant also forms an attachment to its father. They challenged the assumption that the child's preference is inevitably for the mother because she generally feeds and provides more physical care for the child in the early period. [30] Other researchers have agreed that multiple caretakers *per se* are not harmful, provided there is stability and predictability in the child's environment. [26,28,29,31]

It is also important to regard the development of attachment as a

mutual interaction. The mother responds to and learns about her infant while the child is responding to and learning about the mother.
The infant plays an active role in establishing relationships.[32,33,34] An
understanding of the reciprocity of the relationship between the infant
and the caretaker emphasizes that the mother is not the sole person
responsible for shaping the development of a plastic, unformed individual.

While an infant requires availability and consistency, the effects
of sharing caretaking among consistent, responsive individuals must
be further evaluated in this culture. Certainly, it is the prevailing pattern in many cultural settings that a grandmother or older sibling regularly does part of the caretaking.[35] Rutter concluded that

> It seems incorrect to regard the person with whom there is the main bond
> as the most important in the child's life. That person will be most impor-
> tant for some things, but not for others. For some aspects of development,
> the same-sexed parent seems to have a special role, for some the person
> who plays and talks most with the child and for others, the person who
> feeds the child. The father, the mother and brothers and sisters, school
> friends, school teachers and others all have an impact on development. A
> less exclusive focus on the mother is required.[28]

This field of research is relatively recent, and the specific effects of one
caretaker and the critical periods when these might be particularly important have yet to be definitively established.

As noted, those who are concerned about the effects of maternal
involvement outside the home often generalize from findings that have
come from studies of maternal deprivation. Not only is maternal employment not synonymous with maternal deprivation, but the day-
care centers chosen in many of these studies as examples of substitute
care have been among the poorest examples of such facilities.[21,36,37,38]
Studies in these centers show that infants reared in inadequate settings without any stable one-to-one relationship with an adult appear
to suffer affective and cognitive deficits. The conclusions from these
data, however, cannot provide automatic condemnation of all day-care
centers or other alternative child-care arrangements. The connection
between the sterile, understaffed institutional environment and the
setting provided by good day care or other arrangements made by the
middle-class working mother with good resources seems remote. In
countries where women are needed for the work force as well as for
desired population increase, a great deal of attention is focused on the
provision of good substitute care, and no adverse consequences have
been reported.

Some studies have begun to address these issues. There have been
reports that the effect of maternal employment is negative in father-

absent families but not in families with two parents, and that observed distress in children in substitute-care arrangements has been eliminated or modified, depending on their familiarity with the substitute-care setting, the consistency of the arrangement, the caring of the parent, and the available relationships with the caretakers and other children in the setting.[9,21,24,30,39,40] Distress levels were also affected by emerging play interests of the children. Other reports have suggested that the cognitive stage of the child and other developmental variables are also important.[25]

In a review of studies of the effect of substitute care on infants, Murray concluded that developmental progress in the infant appeared to be related to the strength of the mother–infant attachment and the level of stimulation in the home, regardless of the setting of the substitute care.[21] Emotional disturbances, however, do appear to result when mothers put very young children in unstable care, especially children who are under 1 year old. Moore found that children who were placed in day care before the age of 1 year showed more dependent attachment to their parents and more fear than those who went into day care later. In comparing all children receiving preschool day care with exclusively home-reared infants, Moore found that home-reared infants were less aggressive and more obedient, docile, and concerned about approval.[41]

Additional evidence suggests that there may be sex differences in the responses of children to maternal employment and day care; boys' development has been reported to be enhanced by a stimulating environment outside the home, whereas girls may benefit more from close contact with their mothers.[36] The interpretation of these data must also take into consideration the age of the children and the values that are implicitly expressed. For instance, there are possible differences in what is judged to be a desirable outcome of personal style for boys as compared with girls. Bronfenbrenner and others have also called attention to the effects on children of the absence of their fathers and of other adults in their families. The absence of their fathers lowered responsibility and leadership in boys. The absence of significant adult presence increased a child's susceptibility to group and peer influences, which may in some cases intensify antisocial tendencies.[42,43,44]

In evaluating these findings, therefore, one must recognize that the reasons for any observed differences between children of working and nonworking mothers are multidetermined. In addition to the work and care situations, children are also affected by the nature of the early mother–child contact, the prior personality characteristics of the mother, her concept of and feelings about her role, and a variety of family variables. Furthermore, these factors also affect her relationship to the child and her decisions about work.

The impact of sociocultural factors, especially poverty, on the lives of families is also an important concern. Bronfenbrenner pointed out that deprivation and poverty interfere with all parent–child relationships, as do social forces that undermine the confidence and motivation of parents to parent. If the mother is already depressed and deprived, full-time employment can further sap her energy.[42] Discontinuity between generations, instability in families, and changing social forms may create such distance between the values and practices of one generation and the next that in effect, in many instances, parents become essentially absent from meaningful participation in their children's lives even when they are physically present.

THE IMPACT OF MOTHERS' WORKING ON OLDER CHILDREN AND THE FAMILY

There is considerable evidence that a working mother has a particularly positive effect on her daughters.[18] The daughters of working mothers were found to be more likely to choose their mothers as models and as the people they most admired. The adolescent daughters of working mothers, particularly in middle- and upper-socioeconomic groups, were active and autonomous and admired their mothers and were not unusually tied to them. For girls of all ages, having a working mother contributed to their concept of the female role as less restricted, and as incorporating a wider range of activities. Their self-concept reflected these views. They usually approved of maternal employment and planned to work when they grew up and became mothers. Unlike the daughters of nonworking mothers, they did not assume that women are less competent than men. These findings were obtained in a period when working mothers were less the usual pattern than at present and represented a less conventional adaptation.

Studies of daughters' academic and career achievements provide additional evidence of the positive effects of having a mother with career interests, at least in relation to their daughters' careers. A number of investigators have found that achieving women and women who aspire to careers, particularly to less conventionally feminine careers, are more likely to be the daughters of educated and employed women.[18,45,46,47,48] Specific data on sons is scant. However, Hoffman found that the working mother feels less hostility and more empathy toward her children, expresses more positive affect toward them, and uses less coercive discipline, although she may be somewhat "overindulgent."[40] Birnbaum studied the attitudes of professional women toward their children and compared them with those of nonworking mothers. She found that the professional mothers experienced greater pleasure in their children's growing independence, were less overprotective, and were less self-sacrificing.[45]

Data on the husbands of working women indicate that they are more actively involved in the care of the children and that the active involvement of the father has a positive effect on both male and female children.[43,49] Furthermore, the husbands of professional women are more likely to respect competence and achievement in women.[5,18,45,46,47,48,50,51,52]

CONCLUSION

Clearly, there is much to explore in this area, and there are many ways of understanding the processes of family and individual development in a new context. Research needs to be done from an interdisciplinary perspective, and new strategies must be developed for understanding the complex questions of the relationship of early and late development and all the variables in the family and social context. It is clear that we cannot succeed in elucidating processes and influences on development without studies that attend to the realities of people's lives. Thus, it is important to learn about the adaptation of children of single, divorced, and widowed parents and those who must work if we are to take an approach that facilitates success rather than studying only situations predicting failure.

Negative views about the impact of working mothers on their children, such as those implied by Fraiberg, not only perpetuate the confusion between separation, deprivation, and working but fail to suggest realistic alternatives, especially when women have to work.[53] This view also fails to consider the positive implications of the sense of satisfaction and creativity that may be present in working mothers and thus may have an important impact on their children.[54]

Some of the dilemmas faced by women who work are illustrated by Mary Y:

> Mary Y is a 27-year-old divorced woman with two children, ages 3 and 5. She had tried to sustain a marriage to a gentle, warm, but very passive man, who developed a drinking problem a few years after their marriage. An affair he had with a good friend of hers precipitated their divorce. He refused to support her or the children, and after many court battles in which she felt demeaned, she decided that the expectation that he would provide reliable financial support was unrealistic and that it was best to find alternatives.
>
> She was then faced with the problem of finding a job. Although she

was a capable woman, she had married early and had not finished high school. Her family was unable to provide much help. With considerable ambivalence, she took a clerical job and arranged a complicated system of day care and baby-sitters. Her 3-year-old son found the separations difficult and cried daily when she left. She felt guilty, depressed, and lonely. She missed the daily rounds of contact and interaction, which looked very enriching in retrospect. The 5-year-old child was in kindergarten in the morning and then joined his brother. Despite these conflicts, Ms. Y found that the new contacts, the growth of her skills, and her consciousness of her organizational competence helped alleviate her depression, and she began to feel a new sense of strength in herself.

Then, one afternoon, her younger son fell in the day-care center and broke his wrist. She met him in the emergency room of the hospital, where someone from the center had brought him. He was frightened and angry because she had been unavailable. Her guilt mounted. She wondered whether the supervision in the center was adequate. She felt that she needed to change her work so that she could be home more during the day.

With her limited skills, there were few jobs available. She took a job as a waitress, which meant that she could work in the evenings and have a baby-sitter when the children slept. For a while, this seemed a better solution, although she was often tired after returning late and arising early with the children.

The following year her other son entered first grade. He began to stay up later and to ask for help with reading and arithmetic. She felt that he needed more than the baby-sitter could offer. She then chose a different day-care center and again shifted to a secretarial job at a school. The hours made it possible for her to be home early. The salary was less, but she felt more comfortable with the arrangement. However, the work was demanding, the boss was difficult, and the time she had to herself or to explore new relationships was minimal. A friend encouraged her to extend the day-care period, despite the expense, so that she could have some time to satisfy her own needs. With considerable hesitation, she did so, finding to her surprise that the extra hour contributed to making her less irritable. It enabled her to market without having to be accompanied by hungry, demanding children, and then she began to think about an afternoon course.

The continual balancing of needs, time, and arrangements made Mary Y. vulnerable to criticism and evoked guilt. Her ambivalence interfered with fulfillment both in work and in parenting. Nevertheless, for this woman, the gains from some sense of financial independence, from working, and from social interaction were extremely important, and there was no clear solution that did not include some cost. No family situation provides an isolated area of difficulty. Rather, it is the interaction of the parts that eventually leads to the least detrimental alternative for all.

REFERENCES

1. Pifer A: Women and working: Toward a new society. *Urban and Social Change Review* 11:3–11, 1978.

2. Moroney R: Note from the editor, *Urban and Social Change Review* 11:2, 1978.
3. Lozoff M: *Changing life styles and role perceptions of men and women students.* Presented at Women: Resource for a Changing World, Radcliffe College, Cambridge, Mass., April 1972.
4. Katz J: *Past and future of the undergraduate woman.* Presented at Radcliffe College, Cambridge, Mass., April 1978.
5. Rapoport R, Rapoport R: *Dual career families.* Middlesex, England, Penguin Books, 1971.
6. Rapoport R, Rapoport R: *Dual career families reexamined.* New York, Harper, Colophon, 1976.
7. Pearce D: The feminization of poverty: Women, work and welfare. *Urban and Social Change Review* 11:28–35, 1978.
8. Bardwick J: *Psychology of women.* New York, Harper & Row, 1971.
9. Johson F, Johnson C: Role strain in high commitment career women. *Journal of the American Academy of Psychoanalysis* 4 (1):13–36, 1976.
10. Rossi A: Family development in a changing world. *American Journal of Psychiatry* 128 (9):1057–1066, 1972.
11. Campbell A, Converse P: *The human meaning of social change.* New York, Russell Sage Foundation, 1972.
12. Verhoff J: *Psychological orientations to the work role: 1957–1976.* Presented at the Radcliffe Pre-Centennial Conference, Radcliffe College, Cambridge, Mass., April 1978.
13. Holmstron LL: *The two career family.* Schenkman, Cambridge, 1972.
14. McIntire W, Nass G, Battisone D: Female misperceptions of male parenting and expectances, *Youth and Society* 6:104–112, 1974.
15. Bailyn L: Career and family orientations of husbands and wives in relation to marital happiness, *Human Relations* 23:97–113, 1970.
16. Bailyn L: Family constraints on women's work, *Annals of the New York Academy of Sciences* 208:82–90, 1973.
17. Nadelson C, Notman M: Medicine: A career conflict for women, *American Journal of Psychiatry* 130 (10):1123–1127, 1973.
18. Nye FI, Hoffman L: *The employed mother in America.* Chicago, Rand McNally, 1963.
19. Howell M: Employed mothers and their families. I, *Pediatrics* 52 (2):252–263, 1973.
20. Howell M: Effects of maternal employment on the child. II, *Pediatrics* 52 (3):327–343, 1973.
21. Murray A: Maternal employment reconsidered: Effects on infants, *American Journal of Orthopsychiatry* 45 (5):773–790, 1975.
22. Al-Timimi S: *Self concepts of young children with working and non-working mothers.* Doctoral dissertation, Peabody College, 1976.
23. Warshaw R: *The effects of working mothers on children.* Doctoral dissertation, Adelphi University, 1976.
24. Cox M: *The effects of father absence and working mothers on children.* Doctoral dissertation, University of Virginia, 1975.
25. Marantz S, Mansfield A: Maternal employment and the development of sex role stereotyping in five to eleven year old girls, *Child Development* 48:668–673, 1977.
26. Bowlby J: *Attachment and Loss. Attachment.* Vol. 1. London, Hogarth Press, 1969.
27. Klaus M, Kennell J: *Maternal infant bonding.* St. Louis, Mosby, 1976.
28. Rutter M: *The qualities of mothering: Maternal deprivation reassessed.* New York, Aaronson, 1974.
29. Casler L: Maternal deprivation: A critical review of the literature. *Monographs of the Society for Research in Child Development,* 26:2, 1961.
30. Schaeffer H, Emerson P: The development of social attachments in infancy. Monograph in *Social Research in Child Development* 29:94, 1964.

31. Moss H: Sex, age, and state as determinants of mother-infant interaction. *Merrill Palmer Quarterly 13* (1):19–36, 1967.
32. Fries M: Longitudinal Study: Prenatal Period and Parenthood. *Journal of the American Psychoanalytic Association 25*:115–132, 1977.
33. Brazelton B, Keefer C: The early mother-child relationship, in *The Woman Patient*. Vol. 2. Edited by Nadelson C, Notman M. New York, Plenum Press, 1982.
34. Lichtenberg J: *Implications for psychoanalytic theory of research on the neonate*. Unpublished manuscript.
35. Whiting B, Edwards C: A cross cultural analysis of sex differences in the behavior of children age 3–11, in *Annual progress in child psychiatry and child development*. Edited by Chess S, Thomas P. New York, Brunner/Mazel, 1975.
36. Yarrow L: Separation from parents during early childhood, in *Review of child development research*. Edited by Hoffman M, Hoffman L. New York, Rand, Soje, Faindat, 1964.
37. Nadelson C: The women's movement and changing sex roles, in JD Noshpitz, *Basic handbook of child psychiatry*, Vol. 4, Edited by Noshpitz JD. New York, Basic Books, 1979.
38. Notman M: *The impact of social change*. Presented at Southern California Psychiatric Society, 1977.
39. Resch R: *Separation: Natural observations in the first three years of life in an infant day care unit*. Doctoral dissertation, New York University, 1975.
40. Hoffman L: Early childhood experiences and women's achievement motives, *Social Issues 28*:129–55, 1972.
41. Moore T: Children of working mothers, in *Working mothers and their children*. Edited by Yudkin S, Holme W. Sphere Books, 1969.
42. Bronfenbrenner U: *Two worlds of childhood: U.S. and U.S.S.R.* New York, Russell Sage Foundation, Simon & Schuster, Pocket Books, 1970. N.Y.
43. Lamb M: Fathers: Forgotten contributors to child development, *Human Development 18*:245–266, 1975.
44. Brown O: Macrostructural influences on child development and the need for childhood social indicators, *American Journal of Orthopsychiatry 45*:4, 1975.
45. Birnbaum J: Life patterns and self esteem in family oriented and career committed women, in *Women and achievement: Social and motivational analyses*. Edited by Mednick M, Tangri S, Hoffman L. New York, Wiley, 1975.
46. Tangri S: *Role innovation in occupational choice*. Doctoral dissertation, Ann Arbor, Michigan, 1969.
47. Levine AG: *Marital and occupational plans of women in professional schools*. Doctoral dissertation, Yale University, New Haven, Conn., 1968.
48. Almquist E, Argrist S: Role model influences on college women's career aspirations, *Merrill Palmer Quarterly of Behavior and Development 17* (3):263–279, 1971.
49. Young S: *Paternal involvement as related to maternal employment and attachment behavior directed to the father by the one-year old infant*. Doctoral dissertation, Ohio State University, 1975.
50. Maccoby E: Sex differences in intellectual functioning, in *The development of sex differences*. Edited by Maccoby EE. Stanford, Calif., Stanford University Press, 1966.
51. Dizard J: *Social change in the family*. Chicago, University of Chicago Press, 1968.
52. Garland TN: The better half?: The male in the dual profession family, in *Toward a sociology of woman*. Edited by Safelios-Rothschild C. Lexington, Mass., Xerox Publishing Company, 1972.
53. Fraiberg S: *Every child's birthright*. New York, Basic Books, 1977.
54. Kenniston K: Book review of "Every child's birthright," *New York Times*, Section VII, p. 1. Dec. 11, 1977.

Chapter 8

Midlife Concerns of Women: Implications of the Menopause

Malkah Notman

Except for the adult stages described by Erikson, adult development has received little attention until the past few years. Recent work by Neugarten,[1,2] Levenson and associates,[3] Gould,[4] Barnett and Baruch,[5] and others has focused attention on the middle years as a time of development and change rather than a static period or one whose major dynamic is toward aging and death.

Defining Midlife

Midlife for women has in the past been defined in relation to the menopause, often in terms of loss. A closer look at actual midlife concerns for women as well as at the menopause and its implications indicates that this is highly questionable.

Most studies of development, including those of the middle years, have had male subjects and have been based on a male model, where development is seen as proceeding linearly through a series of stages, more or less clearly described. Neugarten[6] and others have challenged this "staircase" view of life.

This conceptualization of universally applicable stages has been criticized further as not adequately reflecting differences in social class and historical circumstances. It is particularly inappropriate for women,[5,7] who may be in different role patterns and phases at differ-

Presented at the 132nd annual meeting of the American Psychiatric Association, Chicago, Ill., May 12–18, 1979. Received July 11, 1978; accepted Feb. 16, 1979. Reprinted from the *American Journal of Psychiatry* 136:10, October 1979.

Malkah Notman, M.D. • Department of Psychiatry, Tufts University School of Medicine–New England Medical Center Hospital, Boston, Massachusetts.

ent times because of changing combinations of children, work, and marriage. Further, women's identity and autonomy issues may be resolved only partially in early adult years, then combined with the developmental experiences of motherhood, and then returned to when children are grown. Thus, the Eriksonian sequence of autonomy, identity, intimacy, and generativity does not hold in quite the same way for women, for whom a more simultaneous development through these phases has been postulated by Gilligan and myself.[8]

Chronological age as a basis for developmental stages has also received considerable criticism.[2,9] For instance, Neugarten,[1] in a study on "the awareness of midlife," found that in a sample of 100 middle-aged "well placed men and women," chronological age was a less important marker for this group than for young or old people. The author noted that the women in this group but not the men defined their age status "in terms of timing of events within the family cycle. For married women, middle age is closely tied to the launching of children into the adult world, and even unmarried career women often discuss middle age in terms of the family they might have had." However, these concepts may be changing in the light of current developments in family patterns.

Levenson and associates' conceptualization of life stages observed in their studies of men[3] gives central importance to the role of work in establishing oneself in the world. Although the importance of family relationships for the adult man is acknowledged, they are not the organizing theme of his life. Separation from the family of origin is placed more centrally in a man's development than is the birth of his first child.

Defining middle age is a complex problem. The central theme in the awareness of midlife for each person seems to be connected with the sense of the finiteness of time left to live in contrast to the infinite perspective of youth.[1,10] For women, this awareness is also closely related to their reproductive potential, and because their lives do take place within the limitations of this biological timetable, the reproductive milestones have been stereotyped as being the central and dominant ones. Although hormonal and physical changes mark the major periods of a woman's life, the characteristics and experiences of these periods may be less related to the actual biological changes and more to social and psychological events than has been assumed.

It is important here to distinguish a woman's concerns about her potential for having children as a framework for her sense of life phase from the idea that her fulfillment and self-realization are limited to childbearing or dominated by children. In reality, many women have not found their children or their role as mothers predominantly gratifying. Children may be draining, stressful, and conflict-producing. However, the finiteness of the period during which pregnancy is possible makes the choice an issue that can not be ignored.

The separation of the biological and social life cycles in recent years has meant that the time of childbearing corresponds less to the span of fertility than in the past and may end earlier or start later than is biologically possible. With the advent of reliable fertility control and the increasing availability of work and careers for women, the birthrate has declined markedly. Many women have waited to have children until their careers are established or have chosen not to have children. The increasing spread in maternal age at childbirth—from teenage pregnancy to the growing number of primiparas who are in their 30s and even 40s—means that age and life phases correspond even less.[11]

Neugarten and Datan's idea that middle age in women corresponds to the point of launching children into the adult world[10] and Rossi's definition of middle age as beginning with the ending of the parental role[12] may be less applicable if children are born later in the woman's life or if their birth is spread over a wide maternal age range.

For women who have not had children, there is an age-related crisis of a sort at about 30.[7] For many women, this age symbolizes the transition from youth to middle age and evokes concern about whether they will ever have children. If this seems unlikely, or if a woman chooses not to have children, contemplation of the finiteness of reproductive possibility creates an early confrontation with what is actually a midlife issue.

MENOPAUSE

In this context, we come to a consideration of the menopause. Menopause is defined as the cessation of menses for one year and thus is a retrospective diagnosis. A more appropriate term for this period would be the *perimenopausal years*. During this time, there is a gradual diminution of ovarian function and a gradual change in endocrine status.[13] Menopause has been considered a dominant factor in the midlife phase of women and blamed for much symptomatology. In clinical discussions of women with depression or other problems, there has been a tendency to focus automatically on the menstrual history as if it constituted an adequate explanation of the symptoms. In fact, the relationships are neither inevitable nor clear.[14,15] Many misconceptions have existed about the nature and extent of menopausal symptoms, and research in this area has been both sparse and poor. McKinlay and McKinlay,[16] in a review of the menopause literature in 1973, and Parlee in 1976[17] pointed to the lack of attention to menopause in the medical literature and criticized the research that does exist. They cited methodological problems such as the failure to develop consistent objective definitions of menopause and of menopausal symptomatology; the use of retrospective data, case histories, and clinical impressions; and the selection of samples from populations of women who are under the care of gynecologists or psychiatrists. The more reliable studies show that "psychosomatic and psychological complaints were not reported more frequently by so called 'menopausal' than by younger women."[15]

This lack of correspondence between symptomatology and endocrine status has been cited also by Perlmutter,[13] who concluded, "There are multiple disorders that have been ascribed to the changing hormonal balance and are equated with menopause. In reality, not all of those changes that are noted are due to hormonal imbalances." Some are the consequences of aging and others have a basis in psychological factors and life patterns.[13]

Age at menopause ranges from the late 30s to the middle or even late 50s. This variation supports the tendency to assign a variety of symptoms occurring during these years to a woman's menopausal status. In a study of age at menopause, McKinlay and associates found that

> The median age at menopause in industrial societies now occurs at about fifty years of age and there is no firm evidence that this age has increased at least in the last century, nor any indication of any close relationships between the age at menopause and the age at menarche or socioeconomic status. . . . There is some evidence that marital status and parity are related to the age at menopause, independently of each other.[18]

MIDLIFE AND MENOPAUSAL SYMPTOMS: UNDOING STEREOTYPES

What symptomatology is directly attributable to the menopause? Vasomotor instability—manifested as hot flashes, sometimes called *flushes,* and episodes of perspiration, sometimes particularly noted at night—is one of the most consistent symptoms accompanying menopause[19] and is present in up to 75% of women who report some degree of symptomatology. McKinlay and associates,[15] in a review of symptoms of women aged 45–54 in the London area, found that hot flashes and night sweats are "clearly associated with the onset of a natural menopause and that they occur in a majority of women." The other symptoms investigated, "namely headaches, dizzy spells, palpitations, sleeplessness, depressions, and weight increase, showed no direct relationship to the menopause but tended to occur together."

The length of time a woman experiences hot flashes is variable. They may originate several years before actual menopause and can be considered a sign of waning estrogen levels. Hot flashes reach a peak at about the time of the actual cessation of the menses and persist for as long as five years.[19]

The etiology of the hot flashes is unclear; they appear to be related to hormonal imbalance rather than simple estrogen deficit. Psychological factors such as anger, anxiety, and excitement are considered important in precipitating flashes in susceptible women, as are activities giving rise to excess heat production or retention, such as a warm environment, muscular work, and eating hot food.[19] However, the symptoms may arise without any clear psychological or heat-stimulating mechanism.

Many other midlife symptoms have been attributed to menopause, and many menopausal symptoms have been attributed to estrogen deficiency or hormonal changes. The symptoms have included insomnia, irritability, depression, diminished sexual interest, headaches, dizzy spells, and palpitations. Neugarten and Kraines[20] studied 100 women aged 43–53 by using menstrual histories as an index of menopausal status. They found "climacteric (menopausal) status to be unrelated to a wide array of personality measures." They also found there were few important and consistent relationships between the severity of somatic or psychosomatic symptoms and personality or test scores. Kraines (cited in reference 14) found that menopausal status did not contribute significantly to self-assessments of middle-aged women. She also found, as one might expect, that women who had had low self-esteem and life satisfaction were likely to have difficulties with menopause. This supports understanding menopause as one of the important experiences for women but one best understood in the context of their entire lives.

Benedek[21] and Deutsch[22] held that a woman's reaction to menopause was similar to her reactions to puberty and pregnancy, although they and others conceptualized menopause as being a loss rather than a change. Deutsch[22] spoke of the menopause as constituting a "narcissistic mortification that is difficult to overcome" and noted that the woman at menopause "loses all she received during puberty." She wrote that mastery of the psychological reactions to this organic decline is one of the most difficult tasks of a woman's life. Deutsch saw increased postmenopausal activity of women as a "struggle to preserve femininity." Femininity in turn was closely tied to sexual attractiveness and reproductive possibilities, according to Deutsch.

This is an expression of a defensive view of femininity, held by many earlier theorists, based on the view that feminine identity is derived from and associated with compensation for something which is missing or "different" about women. In this view, when reproductive possibility is gone a woman must compensate for the loss rather than progress to a developmental stage that is normal for a later period in life. The postmenopausal decreases in estrogen levels can be considered normal for this age, just as low estrogen levels are appropriate for the prepubertal girl.

Benedek[21] believed menopause was a difficult time of complex and demanding personal and social tasks in adapting to grown and more independent children, changing sexual relations with husbands, and changing responses to the woman's life. She believed that women experienced different levels of stress and thought that women who had not borne and mothered children and who were less "feminine" had greater problems. However, she thought that the energy released by the ending of reproductive tasks gave women with flexible egos impetus for learning and socialization.

DEPRESSION AND MENOPAUSE

Depression has been linked with menopause but appears to be more clearly associated with psychosocial variables than with endocrine changes, although depression does constitute an important clinical entity.[23] Weisman and Klerman[24] concluded that the pattern of relationship between endocrine levels and clinical status is inconsistent and that there is good statistical evidence that menopause does not increase rates of depression. Other authors agree[15,23,25] and cite the lack of studies using modern endocrinological methods that have shown correlations between clinical state and endocrine state.

Data from a study by Bart and Grossman[14] indicate that women who have had children, who have "high motherliness" scores on psychological scales, and who have invested heavily in their childbearing and rearing are more likely to experience depression. These findings are opposite to the predictions of both Deutsch and Benedek. Actually, women who have not had children do not always have the most difficulties at menopause. My clinical experience indicates that many women have come to terms with their childlessness before the biological menopause and have found other ways of organizing their lives. The menopause then represents a less critical event. Childlessness may represent the expression of underlying ambivalence about motherhood, which is more readily acted on in contemporary society with less conflict than was possible earlier and can be better implemented with effective contraception and abortion.

Social class is an important variable in the experience of menopause. Middle-class and upper-class women appear to find the cessation of childbearing more liberating because more alternatives are open to them than to women of lower social status. Neugarten and Kraines[20] reported that upper- and middle-class women tend to minimize their reactions compared with lower-class women. In this relatively advantaged group, younger women anticipating menopause were more concerned than women who were actually menopausal. Postmenopausal women generally took a more positive view than premenopausal women, with greater numbers stating that the menopause created no major discontinuity in their lives. Those women who thought they had a relative degree of control over their symptoms felt they did not inevitably have difficulties.

Other studies (reported in reference 14) confirm that middle-class women are less anxious about the menopause than lower-class women but found that across classes menopausal status generally is not associated with measurable anxiety.[19] Bart and Grossman[14] stressed the role of cultural factors in determining the importance of menstruation, child rearing, and mothering in the self-esteem and status of women, as well as in determining their alternatives. Cross-cultural studies indicate that in those cultures where there is improved status at middle age and a clear role for the middle-aged woman, there are greater feelings of well-being in the menopausal years. In our society, women whose lives have not been child-centered and who are still married and women whose children remain close and gratifying have an easier time at middle age and menopause. A woman who has given all of her life to her children and then feels useless when they are gone is more likely to become depressed.

FAMILY EXPERIENCES AND RELATIONSHIPS

Family experiences are important in determining the outcome of this period. The midlife transition for men, many of whom are married to menopausal women, is accompanied by new stresses and often by sexual problems, which can lead to affairs, marital disruption, and abandonment of wives. Adolescent children may be sexually and aggressively provocative, challenging, or disappointing. Children leaving home for school or marriage change the family balance in a way that has been described generally as loss. However, some women view this as an extension and expansion of parenting to include the wider interests and loci of their children. Change and transition do cause stress and require new adaptations, which are sometimes accompanied by symptoms. Studies of marriage[26] indicate that at least in some dimensions, marital satisfactions increase as children leave the home;

thus the "empty nest syndrome" does not seem universal.[26] Separation (e.g., the ability to separate from children as they move out of the family) is an important developmental task at this time. These moves may revive separations in the woman's own past and prove difficult if these separations are unresolved. Occasionally, separation fails and children return, or do not leave. This, too, can lead to depression.

Thus, menopause itself does not appear to be the inevitable source of symptomatology it once was thought to be. However, midlife strains and midlife depression are real clinical entities, and attention must be paid to the social and psychological issues involved. Stereotyping with the automatic conclusions that symptoms are menopausal leads to ignoring the possible help that might be offered and to inappropriate if not dangerous estrogen treatment on the basis of the conceptualization that menopause is a "deficiency disease" rather than a normal progression leading to the next phase of life. There may indeed be some psychological work and even some mourning required before one can move on.

Some women experience this period as being "restored to themselves" and to their own development. This does not mean being alone. Women depend much more than men on maintaining relationships for their development, not only for their emotional comfort and security but also for expressing fulfillment.

The period of midlife has been compared to adolescence. The importance of separation, the change in relationship to family, and the potential for further development of one's own interests are common to both periods. However, the differences are highly significant.[8] At adolescence, the separation is from parents, who are incestuous object choices. At midlife, the separation is from children, and the experience often revives some sense of loss. The adolescent perspective of infinite time and choices to be made differs from the midlife sense of the finite and the reassessment of choices that have been made. The reality is that time is limited and that although choices do exist or even increase, there is also a limited range and variety of careers, new physical pursuits, and new relationships.

CONCLUSIONS

The possibilities for expansion do exist. The potential for greater autonomy, changes in relationships, and the development of occupational skills, interpersonal contacts, and expanded self-image may receive a major impetus after childbearing is over.

Further research is needed about adult development in women in a variety of life circumstances, with fewer preformed assumptions about the phases they are experiencing but with adequate attention to the implications of their reproductive life stage.

REFERENCES

1. Neugarten B: The awareness of middle age, in *Middle age and aging*. Edited by Neugarten B. Chicago, University of Chicago Press, 1968.
2. Neugarten B: Adult personality: Towards a psychology of the life cycle, in *Human life cycle*. Edited by Sze W. New York, Jason Aronson, 1975.
3. Levenson D, Darrow C, Klein E, *et al: The seasons of a man's life*. New York, Knopf, 1978.
4. Gould RL: The phases of adult life: A study in developmental psychology, *American Journal of Psychiatry* 129:521–531, 1972.
5. Barnett R, Baruch G: Women in the middle years: A critique of research and theory, *Psychology of Women Quarterly* 3:187–197, 1978.
6. Neugarten B: Time, age, and the life cycle, *American Journal of Psychiatry* 136:887–894, 1979.
7. Notman M: Adult life cycles: Changing roles and changing hormones, in *Gender roles: A dialectical biopsychological perspective*. Edited by Parsons J. Washington D. C., Hemisphere Publishing Corporation, 1979.
8. Gilligan C, Notman M: *The recurrent theme in women's lives: The integration of autonomy and care*. Presented at the Eastern Sociological Meetings, Philadelphia, February 27–March 2, 1978.
9. Butler R: The façade of chronological age: An interpretive summary, *American Journal of Psychiatry* 119:721–728, 1963.
10. Neugarten B, Datan N: The middle years, in *American handbook of psychiatry*. Edited by Arieti S, 2nd ed, Vol 1. New York, Basic Books, 1974.
11. Price J: *You're not too old to have a baby*. New York, Farrar, Strauss & Giroux, 1977.
12. Rossi A: Transition to parenthood, *Journal of Marriage and the Family* 38:26–39, 1968.
13. Perlmutter J: The menopause: A gynecologist's view, in *The woman patient: Medical and psychological interfaces*. Edited by Notman M, Nadelson C. New York, Plenum Press, 1978.
14. Bart P, Grossman M: Menopause, in *The Woman Patient: Medical and Psychological Interfaces*. Edited by Notman M, Nadelson C. New York, Plenum Press, 1978.
15. McKinlay S, Jeffreys M, Thompson B: An investigation of the age at menopause, *British Journal of Preventive and Social Medicine* 28:16–17, 1974.
16. McKinlay S, McKinlay J: Selected studies on the menopause, *Journal of Biosocial Science* 5:533–555, 1973.
17. Parlee M: Social factors in the psychology of menstruation, birth and menopause, *Primary Care* 3:477–490, 1976.
18. McKinlay S, Jeffreys M, Thompson B: An investigation of the age at menopause. *Journal of Biosocial Science* 4:161–173, 1972.
19. Reynolds S: Physiological and psychogenic factors in the menopausal flush syndrome, in *Psychosomatic obstetrics, gynecology and endocrinology*. Edited by Kroger W. Springfield, Ill, Charles C Thomas, 1962.
20. Neugarten B, Kraines RJ: Menopausal symptoms in women of various ages. *Psychosomatic Medicine* 27:266–273, 1965.
21. Benedek T: Climacterium: A developmental phase. *Psychoanalytic Q* 19:1–27, 1950.
22. Deutsch H: *Motherhood: The psychology of women*. Vol 2. New York, Grune & Stratton, 1945.

23. Winokur G: Depression in the menopause. *American Journal of Psychiatry* 130:92–93, 1973.
24. Weisman M, Klerman G: Sex differences and the epidemiology of depression. *Archives of General Psychiatry* 34:98–111, 1977.
25. Osofsky HJ, Seidenberg R: Is female menopausal depression inevitable? *Obstetrics and Gynecology* 36:611–615, 1970.
26. Bernard J: *The future of marriage.* New York, World, 1972.

Chapter 9

Marriage and Midlife: The Impact of Social Change

Carol Nadelson, Derek C. Polonsky and Mary Alice Mathews

Major social and cultural changes of the past few decades have had an impact on many aspects of life, including marital relationships. There have been modifications in the career, work, parenting roles, and a shift in marital values from an emphasis on survival and economic security to a focus on companionship, love, and communication. A focus on self-fulfillment has superseded more traditional concerns about family integrity. The concept of marriage as an adult partnership between equals, with specific roles and responsibilities, is not new. It is, however, increasingly seen as a partnership between two independent people with individual goals, styles, and personalities.

While much of the recent literature has included discussion of nontraditional marriages, rising divorce rates, and changes in marital sexuality, most of it has been concerned with young couples. We will focus this paper on the impact of social change on midlife couples. We will consider the specific issues of midlife, the factors affecting marital adjustment, and the impact of social change on marital adjustment in midlife.

Reprinted from the Journal of Clinical Psychiatry, Vol. 40, No. 7, July 1979.

Carol Nadelson, M.D., Derek C. Polonsky, M.D., Tufts University School of Medi-cine–New England Medical Center Hospital ● Mary Alice Mathews, M.D. Harvard Medical School and Beth Israel Hospital, Boston.

Midlife Issues

Midlife has most often been defined in terms of age or individual developmental tasks or roles (e.g. the time when children leave home, or the end of the active parental role). These criteria may no longer be applicable, since age criteria vary and the number of people who remain childless or who have their first child when they are in their late 30s and even 40s has increased. Midlife must be defined in more complex terms, which include both individual and interactional criteria, as well as age and role.

The finiteness of time and limited options are inevitable reality issues which must be confronted with varying degrees of psychic pain and pleasure as people grow older. Midlife brings a reassessment of goals and achievements, and a redefinition of roles, with respect to parents and children. This includes role reversal with parents and confronts each individual with his or her position as a member of the "older" generation. In addition, there are multiple separations and losses, including children and friends, which must be faced. The individual must learn to accept the physical changes of aging, which may include decreased capacities as well as illnesses or disability.[1,2,3,4]

Successful adaptation to midlife, according to Marmor, depends upon (1) the integrative capacity of the ego; (2) the nature of interpersonal relationships; (3) the sense of continuing usefulness; and (4) the breadth of outside interests.[6]

On an unconscious level, each person must find a way to accept his or her mortality and resolve the loss of fantasized hopes. Jacques[5] discusses the need to work through the depressive position of infancy again in midlife, in order to achieve a more reflective and philosophical sense of life, as opposed to the optimistic and idealistic views held earlier. If grief work is done, with resignation to imperfections, reparations can be made and generative relationships established.

Recent studies have indicated that while early life problems may be a prelude to later adaptive difficulties, personality changes can and do occur in midlife.[2,3,4,7] Women have been reported to become more assertive and less restricted or guilty, whereas men become more contemplative and nurturing,[3,4] thus reversing traditional masculine and feminine qualities. Although women have classically been seen as more vulnerable to depression in midlife because of the "empty nest," it appears that the major factor in midlife depression in women is role loss when family structures and responsibilities change, rather than the specific loss of reproductive capacity.[8] In fact, the highest incidence of depression in women is not at midlife, but when women are younger and caring for small children.[9]

The difficulties faced by men in midlife are often neglected. Men must begin to integrate their new "feminine" self. They may welcome the opportunity to change, or they may be stressed by this shift in self-image, which requires integrating declining physical powers and decreased opportunities. The implications of the resolution of these developmental tasks and problems for the marital relationship are complex, especially in the context of important environmental changes.

Marital Adjustment in Midlife

In order to understand the process of adjustment in marriage, it is necessary to take account of individual developmental and intra-psychic contributions and, in addition, to view marriage from an evolutionary perspective since "individual and marital development are inexorably intertwined."[10] The conscious or unconscious factors involved in the choice of a mate and the shape of each partner's developmental course and changes, as well as circumstances and environmental influences, contribute to the process of evolution of the relationship. The complexity of the interaction between marital and individual "crisis points" is most apparent at the stage of midlife transition (ages 40–42).[2,10]

The depth of caring and commitment on the part of a couple is tested during the course of a marriage, by the shifts in tasks, expectations, and dynamics which occur. The midlife years bring to a marriage many developmental issues which are similar to those the individual faces. It becomes necessary to recognize and integrate success and failure, and to resolve the loss of the fantasy of infinite opportunity. Priorities in relationships shift away from earlier needs for security, performance, and role fulfillment toward a desire for greater companionship and understanding. This may occur regardless of the particular style of the interaction, level of intimacy, or personality characteristics of the individuals, although these are obviously important.[11] The bonds which maintained the stability of the relationship may be internally generated values, goals, and commitments, relationships with children, and shared activities and interests. At times, partners do not define success or failure similarly, nor do complementary shifts occur simultaneously in each of them. The balance of the relationship may shift, leading to reequilibration and/or adaptation on another level; or the lack of synchronous change may cause the relationship to be strained or disrupted. A change from the original marital "contract" produces stress unless it is mutually acceptable.[12]

Burgess and Wallin[13] surveyed couples married up to 20 years and reported a general drop in marital satisfaction and adjustment, a loss of intimacy, less physical affection, and a decrease in sexual intimacy and sharing of activities at this time. Others confirm these data and emphasize that marital interaction is at its lowest point when adolescents are in the process of being "launched."

The necessity of coping with the parenting demands of adolescents has frequently been cited as a major factor in marital adjustment during midlife. The pain of separation and the necessity of assuming new roles and giving up old ones, as well as the revival of early developmental issues for each partner, are important stresses.

Those who have not had children must also come to a resolution of this as an immutable fact. Depending upon the success with which they have adapted they may or may not be comfortable with the implications of their childlessness.

Furthermore, confrontation with the inevitability of aging may be particularly difficult. Chilman[19] reported that children bring mounting pressure and stress to a marriage as they get older. She described two low points in marital satisfaction, at 7 years and again at 16 years of marriage. These correlated with the stresses of parenting. She stated that midlife parents' feelings of anxiety and helplessness increased when adolescents were most concerned about sexual adequacy and freedom of expression. Adolescent intensity and mood swings may cause parents to feel that the family is deteriorating and may augment their anxieties about their own signs of physical decline and their adequacy as parents and people, as well as missed opportunities, mistakes, and failures.

Couples do, however, frequently express the hope that their marriages will improve and that they will develop greater closeness and companionship after the children are gone.[18] In a review of six national surveys, Glenn[20] concluded that middle-aged women whose children had left home enjoyed greater happiness. These data suggest that the distress manifested at midlife is apt to be temporary. The "empty nest" syndrome was not present for the majority of women, especially those of the upper middle class, where marital satisfaction improved after adolescents left home. This syndrome has been reported to occur more frequently in blue-collar families.[12]

Deutscher[21] studied couples who were in their 40s and 50s with no children at home and defined a "postparental period." He found that these couples valued their increased freedom from the restrictions of time, mobility, financial pressure, and work related to children. He reported that there was a positive redefinition of the individual, and of the marital partnership. The difficulties he cited were those related to (1) the physical disabilities of aging; (2) the pain of self-recognition, particularly if there was a sense of failure either in the work–career sphere or in child rearing; and (3) the inability of some individuals and couples to fill the gap when children leave.

THE IMPACT OF SOCIAL CHANGE

In our current environment, the rapidity of change adds another dimension. The dissonance between the current culture and its values and the world in which most adults grew up creates stress. Many couples have come from "traditionally" oriented families and communities and have internalized those values, despite conscious rejection of their implicit limits. The nature of adjustments and redefinitions which will be required by the social changes of the past decade are not yet clear. We do not know, for example, what will be the impact of dual careers, fewer children or no children, reconstituted families, delayed parenthood or grandparenthood, and changed sex roles on long-term family development and relationships.

What is clear is that adaptation, both in long-held beliefs and values in behavioral dimensions, will be necessary. It is likely that most families will experience divorce in some member, and that single parents and reconstituted families will have to become incorporated into our concepts of family.

Another area, the expanded role of women, which includes that of career person and wage earner, as well as homemaker and child rearer, will require changes in role definitions of men as well. While Clayton has stated that changes in women's roles have occurred without a corresponding shift in men's roles,[16] it is unlikely that this pattern can continue, if the same evolutionary process with regard to roles and relationships continues.

What impact have these social changes had upon couples in midlife? There are few specific data in this area other than the fact that the divorce rate for midlife couples does continue to be lower than for younger couples, despite its general increase in recent years.[22] Clinically, however, there are a number of problems presented by midlife couples which were not seen as often a decade ago. These problems may result in disharmony, if not divorce.

When the evolutionary process in a relationship is disturbed by factors related to social change, as with all disruptive factors, symptoms may appear in one or both partners. When change is viewed as threatening, these symptoms may serve as a cause of seeking help, as a way to effect a separation from a partner, or as an effort to restore a previous state of equilibrium. Symptoms may include depression, anxiety, somatic complaints, and sexual problems. At times, frank and open conflictual issues between spouses, often involving their adolescent offspring, may be presented. Both the form and the content of the problems experienced have been modified by the nature of the adaptations which are necessary in a changing world. These include (1) the adaptational difficulties of a family when the "housewife" returns to work, pursues a career or in some way changes her "role," and changes the equilibrium of the family; (2) the distress of dual-career couples whose goals at this time of life result in their moving in different directions and finding that they cannot achieve their individual ends together without a major compromise by one of them; (3) the changes brought by the birth of a baby in midlife, especially for a dual-career couple who have been childless for a long period of time; (4) the problems of stepparenthood and reconstituted families; (5) nonparallel dysynchronous growth in a couple, especially when it is related to changing values and expectations on the part of one partner; and (6) changed expectations of sexual and other gratifications based on the belief that all of life's offerings must be experienced before time runs out.

While it is clear that aspects of these issues have always been a problem and that they have always caused distress and disruption, they no longer occur as isolated instances. They are part of the fabric

Table I. Presenting Complaints of Midlife Couples

Categories of problems	Number with problems
1. Sexual problems[a]	30
2. Dual-career issues	11
3. Changed expectations (spouse returns to work or school)	9
4. Reconstituted families (Divorce, stepparents)	9
5. General midlife issues (death of parents, retirement, health)	9
6. Failure to communicate expectation (related to roles; individual, marital, parental, or having children)	8
7. Nonparallel or synchronous growth	7
8. Direct response to cultural change (with changing sexual mores, changing societal values)	2
Total number of problems	85[a]
Total number of couples	75

[a]Since couples presented with more than one complaint, the number of problems is greater than the number of couples seen.

of our culture, and few couples will be spared the necessity of adapting to the changing world.

CLINICAL PRESENTATIONS

The case material which follows represents all middle-aged couples who were evaluated and seen either at the Beth Israel Hospital Outpatient Clinic, or in our private practice during the designated three-year period. They have been chosen to illustrate some of the themes delineated above. We have used age as a criterion for midlife in these clinical presentations: at least one partner in the couples selected was past age 35 regardless of length of marriage, number of marriages, or status of children. We will pursue those issues which relate to the influence of social change on midlife couples. Table 1 lists the types of presenting problems in this sample of patients.

Changed Expectations: Adjustment Problems Related to the Beginning of a Wife's Career at Midlife

Mrs. A. was a 40-year-old married mother of a 12-year-old son and a 9-year-old daughter when she resumed her career as a lawyer in a large, prestigious law firm, where she aspired to become a partner. Her husband, a 43-year-old academic, was supportive and enthusiastic. Mrs. A negotiated what seemed to be a reasonable salary and part-time work arrangement. After two months on her job, however, it became apparent that more would be expected of her than she had anticipated, if she wanted to achieve her goal.

Mrs. A felt deceived, and helpless. Mr. A betrayed his ambivalence about his wife's aspirations by his increased demands and expectations. He wanted his life to remain unchanged despite his wife's work, and he was unwilling to make compromises.

Initially Mrs. A blamed her professional field, the firm, and those who made "inhumane" demands. She felt that she was being exploited, and Mr. A agreed. They colluded in their anger against a common enemy. Over the next several months, Mrs. A began to become more angry with Mr. A's unwillingness to participate in family matters or to change his patterns of behavior. She alternately expressed anger and felt guilty when she made even minimal demands, but she would fly into a rage if he did not anticipate a problem and offer to help.

Mrs. A was also unwilling to make any changes in her own self-expectations. She wanted to keep house, shop, cook, and take the children to their lessons as she had always done, but she also wanted to pursue a demanding, time-consuming career. She became increasingly frustrated and depressed but was unable to consider any alternatives. Mr. A, in desperation, sought help when Mrs. A threatened to leave him because he was not "supportive or caring" enough.

Mr. and Mrs. A had clearly made an effective adaptation for 13 years. They had utilized their individual styles and traits in a mutually satisfactory fashion. Mrs. A was well organized and liked to be in control, and

Mr. A wanted her to take care of him while he concentrated on his career goals. Neither partner had seen the obstacles which would arise or the changes which would be necessary if they altered their lifestyle.

The As were very committed to the marriage and cared about each other. They were, however, unable to see alternative "realistic" solutions, and they began to vent their anger, disappointment, and frustrations on each other. They were able, in therapy, to understand their mutual contributions and to recognize the necessity for compromise. Mrs. A began to allow Mr. A to participate in aspects of family life that she had previously believed were her responsibility. She was able to do this without the guilt she had felt when she viewed herself as a "bad" mother. Mr. A was able to offer more, and to see his wife as a friend and companion. He was able to grow toward more independence and at the same time become more nurturant toward their children, without feeling compromised. He became a real support for Mrs. A rather than an obstacle to her efforts to advance her career. At the same time, Mrs. A was also able to examine her work situation more objectively and to make decisions about how far she wanted to go. She was able to make requests for flexibility which both she and her firm saw as reasonable and realistic.

The reentry of the wife into a more active instrumental societal role is often a source of tension and conflict within each partner as well as between the partners, especially when ambivalence is experienced by both partners, along with the enormous potential for disruption imposed by a change in the system. It is important for the therapist to facilitate sharing of anticipated rewards as well as problems. It is often too simplistic to see only the sacrifices necessary. In treating a couple like the As, the therapist must be aware of the realities generated by the world in which they live, as well as those generated by their personality styles, their modes of adaptation, and the defenses of each partner. The therapist must also avoid imposing his or her values and must be able to support those of the couple.

Dual Career Issues: Job, Status and Career Conflicts

Dr. B was a 46-year-old scientist with a tenured university faculty position. Her husband, Mr. B, was 45 and approaching the upper management level of his company. He was offered a promotion if he relocated. Dr. B protested, stating that there was no comparable position for her in her field, and that it might mean the end of her career. Mr. B was angry. He resurrected many previously buried issues, complaining about her lack of interest in his career, her higher income, and his many sacrifices for her. He accused her of being "castrating, selfish, and uncaring." Dr. B felt devastated and deceived. She had believed that they had made a good adaptation, and she had always been gratified by her husband's sense of internal security and his support of her.

There was no solution that did not require considerable compromise and sacrifice, for either or both of them. It was difficult for them to find a way to resolve these conflicting issues. Mr. B expected a reward for his previous compliance, and Dr. B was not consciously aware of his current or past feelings. There had been no mutual or explicit communication to facilitate negotiation.

Mr. B's arguments prevailed, and the family moved. Dr. B obtained a laboratory research position, which offered neither the challenge of her previous job nor the opportunity to be creative. She became increasingly frustrated and withdrawn from her husband and children. Within six months she entered therapy. She was tearful and insecure, feeling hopeless, worthless, and full of helpless rage. The move and the attendant loss of her job and status had been a major stress, which she was unable to resolve.

During the marriage, Mr. B had seen only his wife's competence; he had been unable to appreciate her vulnerability. On the other hand, Dr. B had not been aware of Mr. B's resentment and his shaky self-esteem.

They were each seen in individual therapy as well as couples therapy. In the couples work, they reaffirmed their friendship and love and began to work toward a new adaptation. Dr. B decided to seek additional training in order to advance into a position she had initially rejected because she felt unqualified, and Mr. B was promoted. Their marriage survived.

This situation is often seen in reverse, where the woman has a job offer or career opportunity elsewhere and meets with resistance from her spouse. In either case, the double standard is a significant problem. Traditional values and expectations have required that the woman make the adjustment. Often she, her husband, and the therapist share this view and collude in seeking this solution. These problems test the strength of commitments and, because of the nature and strength of the underlying feelings, provide a potential for destruction of relationships.

The Failure to Communicate Implicit and Explicit Expectation: The Decision to Have Children

Mr. and Mrs. C were a newly married couple who presented with a sexual complaint: Mrs. C had lost interest in sex shortly after they had married. Mr. C was a 50-year-old business executive who had a 16-year-old daughter by a previous marriage. Mrs. C was a 37-year-old nursing administrator who had not previously married. During their brief, intense courtship, they had never talked over plans about having children. Thus, when Mrs. C announced that she hoped they would have a baby, Mr. C was surprised and responded negatively. He stated that he had assumed that she planned to continue her career, which was demanding and time-consuming, and that she was not interested in children. He also revealed that part of his attraction to her stemmed from her involvement in other activities, and his belief that she would be more independent and less demanding than his first wife. Mrs. C was angry and disappointed, and she developed sexual symptoms which she did not initially relate to these feelings.

In therapy, when they began to discuss having children, Mr. C pointed out that he believed that a child would compete for his attention and jeopardize his very close relationship with his adolescent daughter. He was also ambivalent about the demands of a young child at his stage of life.

After all, he said, "I will have an adolescent child when I retire, and I will have added responsibilities when I should have fewer." He revealed that he felt insecure about his ability to be a good father. He felt he was frightened to "try again." Mrs. C was resentful that he could not understand her desires, and that he was in control of her future. As they began to share these feelings and to understand each other better, they were less prone to be accusatory, and they became more empathetic toward each other.

They decided to have a child because Mrs. C felt strongly about it, and Mr. C did not want to feel that he was responsible for depriving her of this important part of her life. He acknowledged that he felt "selfish" when he realized how much it meant to her. She, in turn, realized that she had not appreciated the implications for him of having a child. When she had married him, she had been impressed with his maturity and success and had seen him as a man who would care for her and give her what she wanted. She had really not considered his needs, expectations, and vulnerabilities. The Cs experienced a remission of the sexual symptoms shortly after therapy began, without a specific therapeutic focus on them.

It is important to emphasize here, that the sexual symptoms which were initially presented are frequently the "ticket" to therapy because the symptom is specific and troublesome and the underlying cause may not be conscious or apparent. The therapist must be able to clarify the etiology of symptoms and make recommendations for treatment which the couple can accept. These may include sexual therapy, marital therapy, individual therapy, etc.

A Reconstituted Family: The Problem of Becoming a Stepparent in Midlife

Mr. and Mrs. D had been married for two years. Mr. D had two sons, aged 11 and 14, by his first marriage. He was 46 years old and well settled in his career as an artist. Mrs. D, a 42-year-old editor, had been married briefly and divorced 20 years before. She had no children.

Mrs. D was jealous of Mr. D's attention to his sons. She also complained that he was too lenient and failed to set appropriate limits with them. Mr. D felt guilty about having left his sons. In order to "make it up to them," he failed to make any demands on them when they visited. Mrs. D saw this as a constraint on her and a parenting failure on the part of Mr. D. He was unwilling to discuss this and reminded her that she did not understand how to raise children because she was childless. Mrs. D was angered by Mr. D's attitude and by the many expectations which she stated made her a servant to the boys; she complained that Mr. D neither helped nor clarified his view of the limits of her role as a stepmother. In their sessions together, Mr. D complained about the demands of Mrs. D's career, which he felt relegated him to second place, thus "throwing" him back to his children. He was unprepared to compete with her career, and she was unwilling to make any concessions.

Both of the Ds were strong, successful people, who had each functioned autonomously. They had difficulty learning to listen, to respect their differences, and to accept that part of their commitment to each other which necessitated that each relinquish some control. Neither of them could understand the other's perspective. They both used threats, coercion, and withdrawal of affection when they felt misunderstood. Neither of them had expected that the marriage would bring the necessity of changes and com-promises. In addition, they had not considered the complexity of the rela-tionship between stepparents and stepchildren and the necessity for role definition.

The therapy, directed toward an exploration of goals and expectations, was stormy and difficult because neither partner was certain that the mar-riage was worth the compromises it necessitated. Their commitment to each other was tenuous, and the strength of their feelings was not enough to sustain the relationship. The Ds decided to separate after six months of therapy. They handled the separation without acrimony and with a better understanding of each other and of what they each had brought to the relationship.

The view that marital separation is treatment failure can be an oversimplification of the therapist's values or disappointment. Treat-ment can facilitate the process of assessing the nature of a relation-ship, the commitment of the partners, and the costs of the compro-mises which may be necessary. For many couples, separation may be a better solution than continued belligerence and anger.

Nonparallel Growth in a Marriage

Mrs. E, a woman in her early 40s, came to treatment after her husband had threatened to leave her in order to live with another woman. The Es had been married for 20 years and had three teenage children. For many years, Mr. E had had numerous sexual affairs. Mrs. E knew about them but felt that she simply had to accept the situation because she could see no alternative. She saw herself as dependent and unable to support herself or to be alone.

Initially, in therapy, it was difficult for her to cope with the loss of her husband and she blamed herself for the marital failure. As the therapy proceeded, she began to explore why she had avoided recognizing her dis-satisfaction with the marriage. She became increasingly aware of her anx-iety about independence, and she was able to develop greater self-confi-dence. She recognized that when Mr. E left, she had experienced some relief, as well as anxiety. It gradually became clear that the marriage had been contracted as a way of separating from her family, without working through the developmental issues of adolescence. By marrying, she both left home and remained dependent.

After the separation, when Mrs. E found a job, Mr. E reacted with panic. He wanted to return to her immediately. Mrs. E, however, did not want to reestablish the relationship as it had been, because she felt that she had changed during the period of separation. She wanted to renego-tiate the terms of their relationship so that she could be more autonomous. Mr. E's response to Mrs. E's independence suggested that Mr. E was more dependent on his wife than either of them had believed. Mr. E had been able to avoid confronting his own self-doubt and to take the role of being the stronger of the two as long as Mrs. E complied and was the weaker partner. The balance had remained unchanged until Mr. E decided that he had outgrown his wife. Their separation allowed Mrs. E the opportunity to work through her own separation–individuation issues and to evolve a firmer self-concept. Ultimately, it also enabled Mr. E to confront his own

developmental failure. Conjoint therapy provided a place for them to rebuild their relationship on a more mutually gratifying basis.

At times a temporary separation or a change in direction may initially appear to be damaging especially to one partner, but it may clearly
be turned into a growth-promoting experience. This is especially true
if there are unresolved developmental issues which are masked by
mutual collusion. When the partners can tolerate the anxiety and pain
associated with loss of this collusive balance, growth can occur. A
temporary separation can promote successful resolution of early issues. A similar process also occurs when one partner is involved in
intensive psychotherapy and begins to change. The other partner may
experience this "gain" on the part of the partner as a loss or separation. It is important that the therapist be aware of this possibility when
undertaking individual treatment with a patient who is married.

As expectations and values change in these situations, and individual partners grow, relationships may be strained or disrupted, and
the original contract may need to be renegotiated.[12] This is especially
important when issues of autonomy and self-direction on the part of
a more passive partner begin to emerge in the context of current cultural change.

Sexual Problems Presenting in Midlife

Mr. and Mrs. F were both 43 years old. They had been married for 15
years and had no children. In their first interview, Mrs. F said, "I am frigid
and my husband is impotent." They had not had intercourse for eight years.
They initiated a request for therapy after Mrs. F complained that she felt
that she was missing something in her life. This feeling was precipitated
when younger women at work started to ask her for sexual advice. Mr. F
also agreed to seek help.

The therapist was reluctant to treat the Fs because of the length of time
the symptoms had persisted, and because of his uncertainty about their
motivation to be involved in this potentially stressful treatment program.
Mr. and Mrs. F, however, pressed for therapy. They were treated with
modified direct sex therapy, and within four weeks, they were having sexual intercourse regularly and successfully.

Their feeling that "time was running out" was a powerful moti-
vator. Despite the deeper determinants of their symptom, the fact that
sexuality could be openly discussed made it possible for the problem
to surface, and to be acted upon. For them, the success of the sexual
therapy might, in part, be understood in terms of finally resolving
their conflicts about the procreative purpose of sexuality, with a therapist who gave permission and encouragement in an area which was
previously taboo.

In the past, couples rarely presented with these complaints. The
change in sexual expectations and attitudes has permitted couples to

seek sexual gratification. In our experience, the largest number of couples seeking therapy for a "sexual" problem continue to use these symptoms to avoid acknowledging other marital problems. However, the therapist must be alert to the possibility that treatment of sexual symptoms with available sexual therapy techniques can be successful without long-term marital or individual treatment.

SUMMARY

The special tasks of midlife coupled with the pressures of social change may be highly stressful and may produce symptoms of distress. Renegotiation and restabilization of relationships may be necessary. The fact that divorce is more frequently seen as a solution to conflict makes it even more critical that therapists work with patients toward realistic assessments of the consequences of this solution. The pain of loss of the marital relationship at midlife may be magnified by the many losses which characteristically occur during this life stage. For some, however, the loss of an ungratifying relationship may be experienced as a rebirth of the self.

We have presented several clinical vignettes to illustrate some of the clinical implications of the social changes of the last decade, especially for midlife couples. "Traditional" understanding of marital problems does not address the complexity of these problems. The newly "liberated" woman who has devoted her early adult life to the rearing of children and becomes angry when her husband fails to support her can be understood from a number of perspectives. One can address the issue of her ambivalence about her role as mother or wife, focus on her "low self-esteem" and "excessive need for reassurance," attend to her attempt to master the developmental tasks of middle adulthood, deal with the threats to the husband's self-esteem posed by the change, or view the complexity of the problem from each perspective, recognizing that none of them alone will offer *the* correct answer. The therapist must avoid viewing interactional conflict as unilaterally derived from the psychopathology of one partner.

The change in social values and expectations has also brought changes in the timing of some adult developmental tasks. Couples may become parents later, or not at all; grandparenthood may be a less expectable aspect of midlife, and the prevalence of reconstituted families may bring alterations of family relationships. All of these factors, together with our lack of experience with alternative lifestyles and their impact on families, contribute to the potential for oversimplification and the utilization of conceptual and clinical models which may fail to meet patients' needs. The therapist must be aware of both the contextual and the developmental significance of marital issues at midlife as well as earlier in the history of relationships.

REFERENCES

1. Erikson E: *Childhood and society*. New York, Norton, 1950.
2. Gould R: The phases of adult life: A study in developmental psychology, *American Journal of Psychiatry* 129:5, 521–531, 1972.
3. Neugarten B: *Middle age and aging*. Chicago, University of Chicago Press, 1968.
4. Levenson D: *The seasons of a man's life*. New York, Knopf, 1978.
5. Jacques E: Death and the midlife crisis, *International Journal of Psychoanalysts* 46:502–513, 1965.
6. Marmor J: The crisis of middle age, in *Psychiatry in transition*. Edited by Marmor J. New York, Brunner/Mazel, pp. 71–76, 1974.
7. Vaillant GE: *Adaptation to life*. Boston, Little Brown, 1977.
8. Bart P, Grossman M: Menopause, in *The woman patient: Medical and psychological interfaces*. Edited by Nadelson C, Klotman M. New York, Plenum Press, 1978.
9. Weissman M, Paykel G: *The depressed woman*. Chicago, University of Chicago Press, 1974.
10. Berman EM, Lief HI: Marital therapy from a psychiatric perspective. An overview, *American Journal of Psychiatry* 132:583–592, 1975.
11. Martin P: *A marital therapy manual*. New York, Brunner/Mazel, 1976.
12. Sager C: *Marriage contracts and couples therapy*. New York, Brunner/Mazel, 1976.
13. Burgess EW, Wallin P: The middle years of marriage, in *Middle age and aging*. Edited by Neugarten B. Chicago, University of Chicago Press, 1968.
14. Pineo PC: Disenchantment in the later years of marriage, in *Middle age and aging*. Edited by Neugarten B. Chicago, University of Chicago Press, 1968.
15. Feldman H, Rollins BC: Marital satisfaction over the family life cycle, *Journal of Marriage and Family* 32:26, 1970.
16. Clayton RR: *The family, marriage and social change*. Lexington, Mass., Heath, p. 369, 1975.
17. Luri E: Sex and stage differences in perceptions of marital and family relationships, *Journal of Marriage and Family* 36:2, 260–269, 1974.
18. Thurnher M: Patterns of personality development in middle aged women: Longitudinal study, *International Journal of Aging and Human Development* 7:2, 129–135, 1976.
19. Chilman C: Families in development at midstage of the family life cycle, *The Family Coordinator* 17:4, 297–312, 1968.
20. Glenn ND: Psychological well being in the postparental stage: Evidence from national surveys, *Marriage and the Family* 37:1, 105–110, 1975.
21. Deutscher I: The quality of postparental life, in *Middle age and aging*. Edited by Neugarten B. Chicago, University of Chicago Press, 1968.
22. Bradburn NM, Caplovitz D: *Reports on happiness*, Chicago, Aldine Press, 1965.

Chapter 10

Separation, A Family Developmental Process of Midlife Years

Joan J. Zilbach

> Something very special sometimes happens to women when they know
> that they will not have a child—or any more children. It can happen to
> women who are never married, when they reach the menopause. It can
> happen to widows with children who feel that no new person can ever
> take the place of a loved husband. . . . Suddenly their whole creativity
> is released—they paint or write as never before or they throw themselves
> into academic work with enthusiasm, where before they had only half a
> mind to spare for it.
> MARGARET MEAD, Blackberry Winter: My Early Years, 1972

Recently midlife years have come of age and received deserved and
long-needed attention. The initial quotation is from Margaret Mead's
autobiography,[1] in which she described some aspects of the midlife
years in an enthusiastic and adaptive way. Contrast her statement with
the following:

> Do the observations justify the assumption that normal climacterium rep-
> resents a progressive psychological adaptation to a *regressive* biological
> process? No doubt, adaptation is necessary. There is no other period in
> life—except puberty—when internal changes of the organism put the in-
> dividual's capacity to master those changes to such a test; and while pu-
> berty may be difficult for many girls, even greater is the number of women
> who at the time of their climacteric show signs of stress, strain and *emo-
> tional disturbances* [italics added] of variable severity.[2]

And further,

> The woman [in the climacterium] is *mortified*, because she has to give up
> *everything* she received in puberty.[3] (italics added)

JOAN J. ZILBACH • Director, Family Therapy and Research, Judge Baker Guidance Center, Boston and Senior Training Consultant and Supervisor, Child and Family Program,
Boston Veterans Administration Hospital, Boston.

159

The potential release and the subsequent increase in creative activities and accomplishments described by Mead are also mentioned, although differently, by Benedek:

> It is as if these women, reassured that their main job is done, may draw on the emotional capital invested in that achievement so that they overcome feelings of inferiority and insecurity which inhibited them before. No doubt the emancipation from sexual competition and from the fear of sexual rejection often releases talents and qualities unsuspected before.[2]

At the outset of this chapter, it is important to notice the emphasis on "midlife years" rather than the narrower issues of the menopause or the climacteric that are discussed elsewhere in this book. In these midlife years, there are many biological, psychological, and social tasks that require attention. The biological cessation of menstruation and reproductive capacities that often receive undue emphasis are only two of the many changes and issues that occur in these years. This chapter emphasizes a family developmental and adaptive orientation rather than describing only the pathological and maladaptive complications that may occur in the midlife years.

These differences in orientation are often only implicit in discussions or writings about women. However, they are easy to discern in some popular terms for menstruation, such as the *curse, monthly sickness,* and *falling off the roof.* And likewise, *menopause,* a term that should be neutrally restricted to the diminution and cessation of the menses, has been called a *decline,* an *illness,* a *mortification* (as in one of the passages previously quoted), or *change of life,* which is a euphemism for the cessation of reproductive capacity. These descriptive terms do not immediately imply a potential for both positive and negative changes. The writers of the fifteenth century recognized a period entitled *senectitude* between youth and old age, which was not to be confused with senility. The important characteristics of this period were "wisdom and gravity, not sickness and decline."[4]

Recognizing midlife or senectitude as an important age, we ask what are the tasks of this phase? This chapter discusses the tasks of midlife women in the most important context of their immediate environment, the family. Just as an individual changes over time, following expectable stages of development, so does the family as a collective unit. Every family as an entity, not as separate individuals, has a specific family history with a beginning in time; early, middle, and later years; and an end. Over time, the family as an entity goes through phases of development and the accompanying expectable changes, whatever its particular internal structure. Thus, family development can be distinguished from the developmental life cycles of the individuals within the family. This conception of family life cycles has been

Table I. Stages of Family Life Cycle

Gestational:	Courtship—engagement or other introductory variant. This pre-history affects, in many ways, the early days of the family.
Early:	
Stage I:	The family begins at the point of marriage and/or the establishment of a common household by two people. Family task: from independence to interdependence.
Stage II:	The second phase in family life is initiated by the arrival and the subsequent inclusion of the first child—or the incorporation of another family-dependent member. Family task: from interdependence to incorporation of dependence.
Middle:	Family separation processes.
Stage III:	The third phase is signaled by the exit of a first child or other dependent member from the immediate world of the family to the larger world. This occurs at the point of his or her entrance into an extrafamilial environment. Family task: from dependence to beginning separations and partial independence.
Stage IV:	This phase is marked by the entrance of the last child or dependent member into the extrafamilial environment. Family task: to continue the expansion of partial separations.
Stage V:	This phase comes with the first complete exit of the first child from the family by the establishment of an independent household, which may include marriage or another form of independent entity. Family task: from partial separations to first independence.
Late:	
Stage VI:	Ultimately, the moment comes for the exit of the last child from the family. (This has been mistakenly termed the *shrunken family* or *empty nest.*) It may include the beginning of grandparenthood. Family task: to continue the expansion of independence.
Stage VII:	The final years include the death of one spouse and continue up to the point of the death of the other partner.

termed *developmental family theory.* Although the details of family development [5,6] are not the subject of this chapter, it is important to note that a developmental approach to the family life cycle underlies the material of this paper.

A summary of family development is presented in Table 1 (in each stage there is a phase marker and a family task).

The midlife years of women usually coincide with the middle phases of family development. In these years, individual feminine psychosexual development has as one major task the integration of the cessation of reproductive functioning. In addition, the family as a unit has separate family issues and major tasks in its middle stages.

SEPARATION AS A FAMILY PROCESS

In the earliest years of family life, the boundaries and tasks of a family are fairly narrow, distinct, and cohesive. Over the years, the functions of the family as a unit become more complex and the boundaries widen. In the middle stages (III–V), the boundaries of the family undergo their greatest expansion—to their widest extent. Families may experience this boundary widening as being painful or, at the other extreme, as being an ample, capacious stretching. The middle years of the family life cycle are always complex and demanding. Boundary changes are only one aspect of the family separation processes.

In the course of family development, though one member of the family often is the initiator, all members are involved in the operation and facilitation of the family separation process. The first separation may be the entrance of the first child into the larger community to a day-care unit, nursery, or school. Older dependent members of a family unit may be the first to separate or exit into a nursing home or other institution, such as a hospital. These separations are primarily facilitated by the female head of the household unit, usually the mother, although some are facilitated by other family members with a particular relationship to the separation or exit. Some of these separations are experienced as pleasurable and are viewed with excitement, and others are accompanied by pain. However, the mother is frequently at the center of these events, particularly orchestrating the expression of feelings about the separation. The shedding of a few small tears at the kindergarten door is usually done by the mother and may be acknowledged in words by other family members. The large tear that accompanies the entrance of the last child into the larger world of school and beyond is often hidden. Loss and separation are frequently recognized first by mothers at this later separation from the last child, and family expression depends on the emotional promptings of the mother.

Later in the middle phase of family life, separation events become more distinctly exits from the family. The initial occurrence of a child's moving out to school progresses into the establishment of an independent household unit outside the family, as well as many other more complete separations.

Separation as an important process has been commonly and specifically described as a mother–child issue in the earliest years of life. Thus, separation has been regarded primarily as an early part of the formation of individual identity, which is facilitated by the accomplishment of separation from the mother by the baby. In this chapter, the emphasis is on the importance to women of those separations that are exits from the family as a unit. This process may be experienced in an adaptive, happy fashion or, on the other end of a continuum, as unhappy desertions. These are extremes; in most families there is a mixture of feelings and reactions in the course of the adaptation to these tasks.

Extensive and intensive support is necessary for the accomplishment of these complicated separations. There are many kinds of support: emotional, financial, social, and physical, to name only a partial list. The financial support necessary for exiting children is obvious and is usually recognized. Emotional support is just as necessary. There is often an implicit division of support givers within the family. The father is traditionally seen as the giver of financial support and the mother as the provider of emotional support. Siblings may be called on for physical support, for example, when a family member is establishing a new home. But fragmentation of support is not sufficient for optimal adaptation, and a mixture and interchangeability among family members is more likely to be able to meet the peaks of demand that occur in family life. If an exit is regarded as a desertion by any family member, support is withdrawn by that member, but this withdrawal of support causes subsequent suffering in *all* family members. Since the mother often provides a substantial portion of the emotional support, if she withdraws her share the reverberations within the family are strong.

When the last child leaves the nuclear family, the family unit attains a smaller size, a simpler structure, and different boundaries for the later years of family development. In some instances, the exits from the nuclear family become intermingled with new entrances, into the larger or extended family unit, of grandchildren.

The creative expansion of women at the cessation of their childbearing years is most likely to occur in families that experience the exits as expansions and beginnings, rather than as desertions. In these families, support of many kinds, not only financial, continues unabated and may actually increase during this phase, rather than decreasing. The expansion of the midlife woman is potentiated by the availability of family supports. Men in midlife years also need support for growth in the course of midlife tasks, some similar to those of women and others different from them.

And at the other end of the continuum, families who regard separations in the middle years as desertions feel shrunken, become bitter, and withdraw familial support.

CLINICAL ILLUSTRATIONS

Although the focus of this paper is on normal family developmental processes, the following examples are taken from family treatment
cases in which some maladaptation and/or arrests of family processes
have occurred. Nevertheless, the universal family developmental issues that have just been outlined are illustrated; the family separation
process is emphasized and is seen even more clearly when exaggerated by the occurrence of problems:

> The A family, in Stage IV, consisted of the parents, Mr. and Mrs. A,
> who were both in their midlife years, and four children, ages 14, 12, 10,
> and 8. When the oldest child entered adolescence, serious, intense fights
> between him and Mr. A began and continued unabated. Mrs. A's inter-
> ventions were futile, though all family members exclaimed and agreed that
> these fights were "awful" and should stop. Mrs. A complained of fatigue,
> which became particularly severe after a long, uninterrupted siege of fa-
> ther–son fights. Various individual interventions had been attempted, but
> they had not produced any change in these distressing patterns. Mrs. A's
> somatic symptoms (persistent headaches and fatigue) were considered bi-
> ologically menopausal by her doctor, but estrogen medication did not pro-
> duce relief. Family discussions began and slowly revealed an intense pat-
> tern of nonseparation involving all family members. For example, Mrs. A
> still drove the four children to all activities, with suburban transportation
> difficulties as an excuse. Mr. A quietly supported this pattern because of
> the "importance" of these activities. He felt that his children would not
> complete their projects or studies if their mother did not transport them.
> He did not see taking responsibility by each of them as part of growing
> up; rather, he pontificated about "parental guidance and support."
>   The oldest child's attempts at adolescent individuation and separation
> could be expressed only in ineffectual fighting with Mr. A, whom he saw
> as a possible weak link in the stringent family control of all activity and
> growth. In the ordinary course of family life, in the middle years there are
> many partial exits and expansions, which should occur as little steps to-
> ward separation. Going "away" on overnight visits and trips and to over-
> night camp can be a way of making these partial steps. However, in the A
> family, none of the children had been allowed to be "away" anywhere,
> either to attend camp or to go any other place away from home. Gradually,
> after considerable family therapeutic work, they were allowed to attend
> camps, but only one by one, so that some child was always at home.
>   The parents had been able to establish a household independent of
> Mr. A's parents only after many years of living together, and Mr. A contin-
> ued to work in his father's business. Regardless of the status of the busi-
> ness, and even when Mr. A received offers of outside jobs, the complete
> and unchanged partnership of father–son continued with unabated inten-
> sity.
>   When Mr. A was hospitalized for a "serious" operation, the family
> gathered round and were in constant attendance. This crisis was graphi-
> cally described by family members, who spent many days together in the

hospital, always including all the children. This hospitalization fostered their togetherness, or nonseparation.

Mrs. A was also hospitalized briefly for a tubal ligation described by the family as a "Band-Aid" procedure. The hospital rules were different, so that the children were not allowed to visit, and Mr. A had restrictions imposed, by the hospital, on the amount of time he could visit Mrs. A. These restrictions were troublesome and difficult for this family, and she returned home quickly, with little discussion of the hospital or operation. The issue of the abrupt surgical cessation of reproductive capacity was barely mentioned.

This family experienced many difficulties in the middle phase of family development, especially with the process of family separation. The earlier steps had not been completed.

In the B family, Tom, a 13-year-old boy, began climbing out his window in order to "be with the boys." Discussion with the family revealed that an older sibling, Jim, had recently attempted to separate from the family by attending college away from home. This exit had been unsuccessful, and Jim had left college in the first semester and returned home. He matriculated at the school that his father had attended some years earlier, and he lived at home. As in the A family, the father and the grandfather ran a business together. They explicitly included a third generation, Jim, in their plans for the future of the business, although his inclusion was not particularly realistic from a business perspective.

There were rigid rules about Tom's activities. In essence, they can be condensed to continued pressure to return home and stay. He was officially allowed out only for specific, approved, and time-limited activities. Just "hanging out with the boys" was not approved; that is, the development of increasingly strong extrafamilial, peer relations was a threat to the family. His mother told Tom, "Those boys believe in and do things that I do not like or approve of. If you spend time with them away from home, you will be ruined." His father told him, "You must concentrate on your work and not on your friends." Tom's attempts at separation took the form of defying the rules and making "unofficial" exits through his window. He experienced an increasing inability to study and to maintain his formerly excellent grade level.

The pain and difficulties of separation within the family were clarified in family sessions. After some time, Tom indicated a desire to go away to boarding school. The procedures of finding and applying to a school became a joint family project. After this separation was completed, Tom voluntarily returned on extra visits because he sensed that his mother was lonely and unoccupied. He then helped her make important midlife adjustments. She moved out into the community with his assistance for the first time in her married life.

Although Mrs. B was menopausal throughout this time, she had no significant physical symptoms. Her loneliness was not depression due to menopause but a reaction to the loss of her youngest son. As the entire family was able to face and then succeed in the process of family separation, Mrs. B was able to move out of the house, and her depression abated. She received support from all family members in developing interests and capacities that were not evident in earlier years.

It is interesting that in both of these families there was an inter-generational occupational continuity. While this continuity and inher-itance are a common pattern in many businesses and professions and are not, by themselves, an indication of difficulty in the process of separation, in these two families they were one facet of the way in which the family stayed together regardless of the cost! Over the years, the absence, at various times, of appropriate exits contributed to dif-ficulties in family development.

SUMMARY AND CONCLUSIONS

The middle years of family life are complex and demanding. Dur-ing these years, women face not only the loss of reproductive capacity but the last of a series of exits of children from the family into the larger community. The relationships continue, but first, the separa-tions must be tolerated and even, at times, specifically encouraged. The menopause and the cessation of reproductive capacity are an in-ternal biological event with corresponding intrapsychic changes. The internal sense of feminine worth supplied by reproduction and related activities must be supplanted by other sources of internal worth. These inner reactions of women blend and intermingle with changes occur-ring within the entire family unit during the middle phases of the family life cycle.

Women in midlife are better understood in the full context of fam-ily life and the separation processes of the family life cycle, as has been illustrated in several ways: (1) The mother's fatigue in Family A was not relieved by a recommended tubal ligation. Family problems at that time continued unabated. (2) The loneliness and depression of the mother in Family B were not primarily an internal menopausal reaction but part of difficulty in the process of separation.

There are other important family tasks in the middle years of fam-ily life and the midlife of the parents. This chapter has dealt with only one: the family separation process.

The menopause, an internal biological event in the life of every woman, always has strong individual and personal meanings. Depres-sion may be a result of the loss of the reproductive function, but con-centration solely on internal loss may limit our understanding of mid-life problems and adaptations. The menopause and decline in reproductive capacities are often emphasized as the prime considera-tion for women in their midlife years, and other considerations such as family life are slighted.

But the symptoms of distress in some families experiencing family separation difficulties can be understood more fully when individual and familial concerns are considered together. During these midlife years, families change and some flourish. There are common family developmental issues, including the family separation processes that all families face. A clarification of the family developmental processes, particularly of separation, is useful to women as they confront the stresses and strains on their central role in family life in their own middle years:

> All work and no play makes Jack a dull boy,
> All pleasure and no work makes Jill a dull girl.

And to paraphrase further,

> All closeness and no separations make Jack and Jill and their family seemingly secure but actually stagnating, not quite alive, especially in the middle phases of family life, Stages III, IV, and V.

REFERENCES

1. Mead M: *Blackberry winter: My earlier years.* New York, William Morrow, 1972.
2. Benedek T: Climacterium: A developmental phase, *Psychoanalytic Quarterly* 19:1–27, 1950.
3. Deutsch H: *The psychology of women.* New York: Grune & Stratton, 1944.
4. Ariès P: *Centuries of childhood: A social history of family life.* New York: Knopf, pp. 21–22, 1962.
5. Zilbach JJ: Family development, in *Modern psychoanalysis.* Edited by Marmor J. New York: Basic Books, pp. 355–386, 1968.
6. Zilbach JJ: Family development and familial factors contributing to disturbances of development in childhood and adolescence, in *Basic handbook of child psychiatry.* Edited by Noshpitz J. New York: Basic Books, pp. 62–78, 1979.

Chapter 11

Women and Aging

Golda M. Edinburg

Aging is a poorly understood phenomenon, both physiologically and psychosocially. Our ignorance reflects our youth-oriented society and its massive avoidance of the subject of aging and death. It accounts for the persistence of the many myths, prejudices, and stereotypes associated with the aging process.

The potential for social, economic, physical, and mental changes, as well as the many misconceptions about aging, contribute to its being the most devalued stage of the life cycle by both young and old. When queried about the quality of her life, one woman, age 84, responded that the worst part was being treated like a "decrepit old lady." She did not want to see herself as old and did not want to think about what she would do if she could no longer care for herself; she would cross that bridge when she came to it.

The mounting numbers of older persons—now 23 million—make them more visible and the attendant psychosocial, economic, and political issues more pressing. The elderly themselves are having their consciousness raised and are becoming more vocal and militant in their own behalf. For both humanistic and pragmatic reasons, avoidance and indifference are giving way to increasing attention from clinicians, researchers, government personnel, and politicians in an effort to gain more systematic knowledge of the process of aging in all its personal and social ramifications; to assess the consequences of the demographic shift in the elderly population; and to suggest appropriate individual, familial, and societal responses.

There is much confusion in defining just who the elderly are. Is the question decided on the basis of chronological age or appearance,

Golda M. Edinburg, ACSW • Director, Social Work Department, McLean Hospital, Belmont, Massachusetts.

or because an individual is no longer employable or productive, or because of deteriorating mental or physical health, or because of loss of status in the family or society?

The chronological age of 65 has generally been considered the demarcation point between middle age and old age in conformity with U.S. Census groupings, the frequently mandatory retirement age (before it was raised to 70 in 1978), eligibility for social-security retirement payments (except for women's option to collect reduced benefits at age 62), eligibility for Medicare, and qualification for community services. This is a somewhat arbitrary number, however. As the life span increases, the period of middle age will probably expand as well, particularly with mandatory retirement advanced to age 70. It has been suggested by one writer in the field that the 20 years between the ages of 50 and 70 are the "better half of Middlescence" which is a stage beginning at about the age of 30. "This is the command generation. Practically all people in decision-making positions come from this group—'the new middle age.' "[1]

Those over 65 are not a homogeneous group. Far from it. One must differentiate among those in their 60s, their 70s, their 80s, or beyond; among the married, the widowed, the divorced, or the single; among those who have had professional or nonprofessional careers; who have living children or other relatives or no family at all; who are still working or are retired; who are financially secure or living in poverty; who have been influenced by diverse social, ethnic, and cultural attitudes; who are white or from a minority group; and, most importantly, who are in good physical and mental health or in varying degrees of ill health.

Because of the lengthening human life span, the U.S. population over the age of 65 has increased dramatically, both numerically and proportionally, from 4% (3 million people) in 1900, to 11% (23 million) in 1977, to a projected 15% (31 million) by the year 2000, and to 20%–23% (about 55 million, roughly 1 out of 5) by the years 2020 to 2030, when the cohort of the postwar baby boom will have peaked. Women over 65, because of their greater longevity (a life expectancy of 77.1 years in contrast to 69.3 years for men), are the fastest-growing segment of this aging population; within this group, the proportion 75 years and over is getting larger. Women outnumber men 100 to 79 at ages 65–74 and 100 to 48 at 85 years and over,[2] and the differential is increasing.

Neugarten stated that

> important differences exist between men and women as they age. Men seem to become more receptive to affiliative and nurturant promptings; women more responsive toward and less guilty about aggressive and ego-

centric impulses. Men appear to cope with the environment in increasingly abstract and cognitive terms; women, in increasingly affective and expressive terms. In both sexes older people move toward more egocentric, self-preoccupied positions and attend increasingly to the control and satisfaction of personal needs.[3]

Recognizing role and sex differences, Cumming wrote in 1963 that special theories of aging are required for men and women.[4] The task of drawing such distinctions, however, is hampered by the unequal amount of data (most of the studies in the past have focused on men) and by the undetermined effects of the accelerating changes in women's roles, lifestyles, and self-perceptions. Nevertheless, some sex distinctions in the aging process have been noted, along with many features that are common to both men and women. Accordingly, this chapter presents a broad perspective on the phenomenology and implications of aging and tries to tease out the unique aspects of the experience for women. Case examples highlight the adaptations, maladaptations, and stresses of this stage of the life cycle.

DYNAMICS OF AGING

The phenomenon of multiple loss is a striking feature of the lives of older people and has fundamental significance for understanding the dynamics of this period of life. Along with loss go grief and frequently anger, denial, and depression, which can bring in their wake projection, somatization, alcoholism, etc.—in short, many of the behaviors often associated with aging.

Loss by death of a spouse, siblings, friends, and colleagues occurs with mounting frequency, and as more people live to advanced old age (the proportion of people 75 years and over had increased to 3.8% of the U.S. population by 1975, three times the rate of the people in the 65–75 age group),[5] more of the elderly outlive their adult children. With physical aging comes the continuing loss of youthful appearance, the slowing down of physiological and mental functioning, and the potential for loss of physical health, mobility, sensory perception (vision, hearing, and taste), and memory, all conducive to loss of self-esteem. With retirement come the loss of role identity, possibly a pervasive loss of identity; the loss of structured activities; and frequently the loss of financial security, social status, and, again, self-esteem. Reduced income may necessitate a change in living arrangements and a loss of independence. The possibility of role reversal, with dependence on one's children or others, is frightening and may further reduce self-esteem. Changes in living arrangements and network and support systems require an adaptability and a flexibility not usually expected in an older person.

Actually, adjustment to change is difficult at any age. C. Murray Parkes has addressed this often-observed phenomenon with a conceptualization that aims at linking stress research, loss research, and crisis studies. Major changes, or psychosocial transitions—whether for seeming good or ill—are defined as those changes that

1. are lasting in their effects;
2. take place over a relatively short period of time;
3. occur in the individual's *life space*,* "those parts of the environment with which the self interacts and in relation to which behavior is organized; other persons, material possessions, the familiar world of home and place of work, and the individual's body and mind insofar as he can view these as separate from his self"; and
4. affect large areas of the individual's *assumptive world*,† "the only world we know," which includes "our interpretation of the past and our expectations of the future, our plans, and our prejudices."

As an example, a man who lost his job is deprived of "a place to work, the company of workmates and a source of income," all changes in his life space. Corresponding changes in his assumptive world concern "the way in which each day must be spent . . . , the sources of money and security . . . , his view of the world as a safe, secure place," etc.[6]

An individual is tied to the segments of his or her life space and to the corresponding assumptive world by affective bonds, which by their very nature are resistant to severance and "hence, resistance to change." Grief work, so conspicuous in the lives of older people, is actually the process of restructuring the assumptive world. Advance planning can reduce the stress of change by facilitating the relinquishment of parts of the life space and the restructuring of the assumptive world.

How individuals cope with the changes that aging brings is largely a function of the patterns of behavior and the personality configurations previously established. Personality is continuous over time (although not ossified; at all stages of life, it is subject, in varying degrees, to modification by intervention or by life experience). Those who have been characteristically rigid or dependent or withdrawn will very likely continue to be so; those who have been flexible, indepen-

*A term originated by Kurt Lewin.
†A term Parkes derived from Cantril's "Assumptive Form World" referring to perceptual elements.

dent, or gregarious will continue to manifest those qualities. Older people are as diverse as any younger population, probably more so because they have lived longer and seen more.

The theory of continuity of personality does not mean that massive stress and loss doesn't produce significant symptomatology. Many gerontologists believe that senile behavior is to a large extent socially induced and can be created at any age in anyone who is stripped of role, status, economic independence, and physical well-being.

In order to distinguish between normal changes of aging and pathological processes, it is useful to view aging from the theoretical perspective of a "normal developmental phase of life with its own tasks that can be successfully mastered as were tasks of earlier phases of life."[7] Opposed to this view is the reactive theory of aging, which has emphasized the reactive processes to environmental stress. Butler[9] is a strong proponent of the concept of aging as an inherent stage of the life cycle, in which there is no termination of the potential for change. The developmental concept of aging is exemplified by Erikson, whose eight life stages conclude with late adulthood "maturity," which is the culmination of the acquisition of "ego identity" that began in infancy: "It is the acceptance of one's one and only life cycle as something that had to be and that, by necessity, permitted of no substitutions." The antithesis of ego identity is "despair": "The lack or loss of this accrued ego integration is signified by fear of death. . . . Despair expresses the feeling that the time is short, too short for the attempt to start another life and to try out alternate roads to integrity."[7]

The disengagement theory of aging postulated by Cumming and Henry—that society withdraws from the aging person to the same extent as the person withdraws from society[8]—has been disputed by many. Butler contended that older people who disengage by withdrawing into themselves or choosing to live alone, or exclusively with their peers, are displaying only one of the many patterns of reaction to old age.[9] Charatan stated that it is not clear whether disengagement is voluntary or is brought about by social forces directed at the older person.[10] Havighurst et al. proposed that personality is the pivotal dimension in the various patterns of aging.[11]

BEREAVEMENT

Women are especially vulnerable to bereavement. They suffer losses of friends and relatives, including parents, children, and siblings. Because they outlive men by almost 8 years and are customarily at least 3 years younger than their husbands (sometimes decades, especially if it is a second marriage for the man), they can expect at least 11 years of widowhood, with little chance of remarriage.[12] For women over the age of 65, widowhood is almost inevitable; among those over 75, almost 70% are widows. In contrast, most men 65 and over—three out of four—are married and living with their wives. In addition to the grief and loneliness of bereavement, Weiss found that the bereaved also suffer more sickness, serious illness, and emotional distress.[13]

PHYSICAL AND PHYSIOLOGICAL CHANGES OF AGING

Aging brings changes in physical appearance, beginning subtly in the fourth decade and accelerating as aging progresses, the timetable somewhat variable depending on heredity, diet, and exercise. Good nutrition, sufficient rest, and a program of exercise tone muscles and improve flexibility, protecting the body against injury and disease. Exercise helps to maintain the elasticity of blood vessels, keeping the blood flowing and nourishing body cells and organs. Although exercise may slow down the process, physical and physiological changes still occur. Connective tissue loses its elasticity, muscle tone and tissue diminish; skin dries out, and the face wrinkles; the body becomes progressively flabbier; chin, throat, eyelids, breasts, upper arms, thighs, and abdomen sag; the bones lose minerals, the skeletal frame compresses, and a "dowager's hump" develops; age spots appear, and the hair becomes thinner (most noticeably in men) and loses its color.

The loss of youthful appearance is especially difficult for women. Susan Sontag, reflecting on the double standard of aging, pointed out that physical attractiveness is more important in a woman's life than in a man's.[14] A woman's self-image is inevitably bound up with her physical attributes. To slow down physical deterioration and to combat the narcissistic insult that women experience, Dr. Robert Goldwyn described the increasing acceptance of plastic surgery to counteract the ravages of facial wrinkling and body sagging.[15] Only the affluent can consider this option, however, as most cosmetic procedures are not covered by health insurance.

Added to the visible alterations are changes that affect all areas of the body's functioning. The heart pumps less blood—a decrease of about 8% each decade after adulthood; the blood pressure increases as fatty deposits cause the arteries to narrow; the peripheral circulation is weaker; and the lung capacity is reduced, depriving the tissues of oxygen. Muscle strength and bulk decline and the proportion of body fat increases. Joints stiffen and wear out. Metabolism slows down.

Sensory perception—sight, sound, taste—declines. The immune system is no longer as effective: 1/10 the strength in the 60s as in adolescence. Fatigue sets in more quickly. Emotional responses are reduced. After age 30, the brain loses neurons at the rate of 100,000 a day from its maximum of about 12 billion at maturity. These are not regenerated. Many of these changes are accelerated by physical inactivity and can be slowed down—in some cases, reversed—by a program of exercise, even for the elderly.

It is important to differentiate the normal processes of aging from pathological conditions. For instance, some of the changes usually associated with age, such as cerebral blood flow and oxygen consumption, are also a function of cerebral vascular disease. Contrary to the stereotype of the elderly person, senility is *not* inevitable, nor are confusion and memory impairment. It is true that the body and the mind slow down, probably as a result of the gradual destruction of brain cells; more time and energy are required to accomplish physical and mental tasks, and mild memory loss is common. But these changes frequently do not manifest themselves until the late 70s or into the 80s, and not always then; there are many examples of older people in their 80s and 90s whose minds are clear and keen.

Studies have shown that vocabulary expands with age, and if the person is given enough time to complete a task, cognitive ability shows little decline. Kastenbaum demonstrated that "senile" symptoms could be induced in college students.[16] What started out as a manageable task became complicated and frustrating by simply speeding up the assignment of matching cards. When the students could not perform fast enough, they became angry, jittery, and agitated, just as older people tend to become impatient, irritable, and frustrated as their reactions slow down and they do not take enough time—or are not given enough time—to think, remember, or complete a task. With awareness, sensitivity, and a modicum of effort, the slower reaction time of older people can be compensated for.

SEXUALITY

Despite physiological changes in both men and women, sexuality is not sharply discontinuous, as the stereotype would have it, but follows a developmental course. Postmenopausal changes in women, resulting from lowered levels of estrogen, include a narrowed, tightened vagina (because of the reduced elasticity of the connective tissue) and a drying and shrinking of the vaginal wall that can lead to diminished lubrication and sometimes dyspareunia (pain on intercourse). Most women have mild or minimal difficulty, which is effectively countered with dilators or lubricants.[17]

Both men and women can expect some decrease in frequency of coitus and "reduced *objective* intensity of orgasm" but "sustained and even increased *subjective* enjoyment into the nineties."[18] Sexual pleasure, of course, is not measured only by orgastic release; it includes the whole range of warm, loving, physical contact that can also yield deep and satisfying enjoyment.

Reports from the limited research data available indicate that women are interested in and do have active and satisfactory sexual experiences well into old age. From a sample of 11 women over 60, Masters and Johnson concluded that "regardless of involutional changes in the reproductive organs, the aging female is fully capable of sexual performance at orgasmic response levels, particularly if she is exposed to regularity of effective stimulation.[19] Other researchers[20,21,22,23,24] have drawn similar conclusions. Berezin also concluded that those who are sexually active when young are sexually active when old.[25]

Although the capacity for sexual enjoyment extends into old age, the opportunity does not. Women become sexually ineligible long before men. The higher mortality rate of men, the high divorce rate, and the double standard of aging combine to reduce drastically the availability of peer sexual partners for older women. Widowed or divorced older women are passed over by the tendency of men to seek out much younger women. It is considered perverse if an older woman is sexually involved with a man 20 years her junior, but it is acceptable for an older man to be involved with a woman as much as 50 years his junior. In a study of remarriage probability after widowhood, it was found that remarriage probabilities are high for persons widowed before age 35 but decrease faster for widows than for widowers; for men over 65, the remarriage rate is 5 times that of women over 55. Men also remarry more quickly than women, a median interval of 1.7 years, compared with 3.5 years for women.[26]

PHYSICAL HEALTH

When questioned about what was most important to them at this stage of life, a small sample of women over 60 replied, "good health"; "Thank God I'm well enough to take care of myself"; "I was doing very well until I broke my hip and started to have trouble getting around"; "If my arthritis weren't so painful, I'd be able to do more"; "I'm putting off having a cataract operation because I'm afraid I'll go blind and will need to be cared for"; "I have less strength and can't do as much as I used to do, so I have to plan my days according to my energy level."

These initial responses reflect the older woman's primary interest in the state of her health. Understandably so, as the risk of forced change in the way of life caused by illness or disability increases enormously in the upper years.[27]

In 1973, persons 65 and over (10% of the population) accounted for 28% of the $80 billion spent on personal health care.[28] In 1975, the noninstitutionalized elderly had an average of 6.6 medical contacts per year, and one-third of the average physician's patients were over 65.[29] The older woman consults a physician more frequently than her male counterpart but uses less expensive medical services.[30]

Elderly women, who are on the average older than elderly men, have higher rates of arthritis, diabetes, hypertension, back impairments, and visual impairments; they are susceptible to osteoporosis (excessive calcium loss or softening of the bone), causing low back pain and hip fractures; unexplained attacks of falling down; and muscle spasms. Men have higher rates of asthma and chronic bronchitis, hernias, ulcers, and hearing impairments.[31] Because many older people are depressed and withdrawn, regardless of social class, they may be apathetic about cooking and eating and often suffer from enzyme deficiencies and malnutrition (vitamins are recommended as a supplement to inadequate diets).

Racial factors affect the health of women. In a national survey, 28% of black women, compared with 13% of white women, suffered three or more physical disabilities; 52% of white women compared with 22% of black women said their health was good.

Diseases of the heart are the leading cause of death for both men and women over 65, occurring almost three times as often as malignant neoplasms (cancer), the second of the major causes of death. Women have a higher death rate than men from diabetes and kidney infections.[31]

Unlike medical care, dental services are underutilized by the elderly. The proportion of old persons visiting a dentist is strongly correlated with income, suggesting that dental care is not considered a necessity by many people. This is a serious misapprehension. Half of the elderly have no teeth, and in 1971, 44% of this group did not have properly fitting, useful dentures. In 1960–1962, a large proportion of the elderly who did have teeth (36% of women and 59% of men) had destructive periodontal disease and an average of 18 teeth missing. Adequate dental care has major psychological and health benefits; it stimulates socialization, and it contributes to better nutrition by making eating more enjoyable and enlarging the diet.[31]

A major problem in the medical treatment of the elderly is their increased sensitivity to medication because of changes in absorption, metabolism, and excretion and because a higher proportion of fat cells permits the accumulation of some drugs. What might be considered a normal dosage for a 40-year-old could be much too strong for an 80-year-old and could produce toxic or other serious reactions. Drug intoxication is frequently mistaken for senility. A study done on sleeping pills and released by the National Academy of Science in 1977 showed that drugs such as the benzodiazepenes (Librium, Valium) may aggravate mental and physical conditions in the elderly, who receive 39% of all sleeping pill prescriptions; those with kidney problems are particularly vulnerable. A complicating factor is the multimedication of the elderly: the average person over 75 is on multiple drugs at any one moment.[32]

Perhaps the worst problem of health care for the elderly is benign neglect. All too often, physical symptoms are disregarded by the individual, who wants to deny that anything is wrong, or by a physician, who cavalierly attributes the complaint to "old age" and does not carry out a thorough examination and a subsequent treatment regimen.

In 1979 the median income for elderly women living alone was $4,538, and for men, $5,275, well above the poverty line.[41] Thus, maintaining independent living arrangements is more difficult for elderly women, who are more likely than men to live alone.[29] Frequently, it is up to the children to step in and arrange proper medical and physical care. Some children have difficulty taking on these caretaking responsibilities, rationalizing that their parents want their independence or that they can handle their own affairs.

Frequently, the elderly are misdiagnosed as senile, and their symptoms are given short shrift on the assumption that nothing can be done for this condition. Misdiagnosis sometimes occurs because the elderly respond to physical illness in a different way from younger people. Mental confusion is often the first symptom of many diseases, such as drug intoxication, heart attack, hypoglycemia, malnutrition, vitamin deficiency, renal failure, and appendicitis; depression is frequently mistaken for senility. Many of the early symptoms of dementia differ little, either qualitatively or quantitatively, from those that occur in normal, healthy individuals who are exhausted, anxious, or subject to severe environmental pressures.[33] For example, a 67-year-old widow who, because of financial pressures, is forced to sell her home and move to housing for the elderly can exhibit symptoms of forgetfulness, confusion, loss of appetite, somatic complaints, withdrawal, etc., all of which could be indicative of depression rather than dementia.

Many diseases of the elderly are responsive to appropriate interventions. Stroke victims, for example, demonstrate striking improvement with vigorous rehabilitation efforts. Dr. Robert Gibson reported a survey of 6,400 patients admitted to 40 psychiatric hospitals between 1960 and 1964; 75% of patients over 65 improved and returned to their homes within two months.[34]

Senile Dementia

True senile dementia is a distinct disease process involving organic brain damage. It affects 4 million elderly people, 15% of those in the 65–75 age group and 25% in the 75-and-over group. One type of senile dementia is Alzheimer's disease, for which there is no known cause or cure and which for unknown reasons occurs more often in women than in men—a ratio of 2½ to 1. Symptoms such as memory loss, carelessness, and loss of interest in surroundings may appear insidiously between the ages of 40 and 60 and progress until the person is confused, incoherent, and disoriented.

Multiinfarct dementia, or multiple strokes, affects the arteries of the brain and can also cause irreversible mental changes, depending on the extent of the cerebral vascular accident and the particular area in which it occurs. Symptoms include headaches, dizziness, noises in the ears, lack of concentration, insomnia, and memory defect. As the disease advances, disorientation and delusional ideas develop, with odd behavior and a loss of bowel and urinary control. Treatment of this condition with anticoagulants, vasodilators, and surgery has had some success.

Mental Health

The incidence of emotional illness increases with age, so that 20%–30% of patients over 60 have psychiatric symptoms. Older persons account for approximately one-quarter of new admissions to state mental hospitals and constitute a high proportion of the long-term residents in such institutions.

With deinstitutionalization decreasing the population of mental hospitals, the number of older persons being treated in general hospitals is increasing substantially.[35] According to Shanas and Maddox, 75% of the first admissions between ages 65 and 74, and 49% of those 75 and older, are admitted with the diagnosis of chronic brain disease.

Approximately 10%–20% of those so diagnosed have reversible conditions.[35]

Townsend, studying admissions in Britain, found that the rate of institutionalization for emotional illness correlated highly with sex and marital status. He reported that an unmarried female was twice as likely to be institutionalized as a widowed or married woman. The rate for unmarried men was 4 times as great. Even in nonpsychiatric hospitals, there was a disproportionate excess of unmarried persons.[36] The incidence for men seems to bear out the observation that women cope better with aging than men do. Men need to be cared for because they have fewer of the homemaking skills.

DEPRESSION

Of the main psychiatric syndromes seen in elderly people—depression, hypochondriasis, paranoid reaction, situational disturbance, and alcoholism—the most common is depression, with an incidence of 10% for ages 66–75, declining to 4% beyond the age of 75, perhaps because people with severe depression don't live that long. At younger ages, women have a higher rate of depression, but after 55, men catch up.[12] Depression is frequently associated with a separation or a death or physical illness. Loneliness, social and economic difficulties, a change in living arrangements, an accident such as breaking a hip or leg, or hospitalizations for medical or surgical care can lead to confusion or despair.

Depression in the elderly is often expressed by malaise, fatigue, insomnia, somatic or hypochondriacal complaints, loss of appetite, feelings of loneliness and helplessness, sadness, boredom, alcoholism or drug abuse, loss of sexual drive (impotence in men), and states of forgetfulness and confusion. Because these symptoms may be taken for evidence of organic illness, or overlooked entirely, depression is frequently not recognized by the individual, the family, or the physician. Serious medical complications can ensue, such as poor nutrition's compounding an alcohol problem or liver and heart damage resulting from the drinking. Insomnia and loss of appetite can cause weakness and dizziness, with consequent confusion, unsteadiness, and falling, thus increasing the potential for accidents.

Fortunately, depressions are responsive to treatment. A psychotherapeutic approach aims at understanding and alleviating the cause of the depression; a psychopharmacological approach aims at correcting the brain's biochemical imbalances associated with the depressive syndrome. When properly prescribed and monitored, antidepressants can be highly effective. Caution must be exercised, however, because, as with all drugs, older people are particularly susceptible to side effects and because antidepressants may interact with other medications that the elderly may be taking. For the best results, the two approaches should be used in concert. It is possible that under some circumstances, the identification and alleviation of situational stresses can relieve the depression; when medication is indicated, it should *always* be accompanied by psychotherapeutic intervention to assist the patient in replacing lost object relationships, activities, living situations, etc.

The following case illustrates a typical example of depression in women, regardless of age, marital status, or socioeconomic background:

Depression in a Married Woman

Ms. Green, age 65, was hospitalized for agitation and depression after she had overdosed on sleeping pills. She related her upset to her concern about her youngest daughter, who was embroiled in a bitter divorce battle. Ms. Green had become critical of and impatient with her daughter. She overreacted and began to withdraw; she stopped eating and was having trouble sleeping. She felt that her husband, who was about to retire from the post office, was harassing her because she was so weak. Mr. Green, in turn, was worried about limited income on his retirement. Between fears about his future and his resentment of his wife, he had become impotent. Ms. Green felt responsible for his impotence and was sexually frustrated. She then felt even more worthless and unimportant. She had had two previous periods of depression: first, when her mother had died 30 years before, and then when her favorite daughter had married and moved away from home 10 years before. She had responded well to antidepressants during both past episodes and quickly recompensated on resumption of the medication. During the hospitalization, both husband and daughter spoke of their concern about Ms. Green's vulnerability to tensions in the family. They also acknowledged that their own worries about themselves lowered their tolerance and acceptance of her needs. As the daughter reviewed her complaints about her mother, she could see that many of the issues stemmed from her own internal responses to her marital alienation. She decided to seek therapy for herself. Mr. Green, in reviewing his reactions and concerns, felt that he was being unnecessarily hard on his wife as a result of the pressure he was undergoing himself. He and Ms. Green both felt that joint meetings with a therapist could help them work out the tensions in themselves and in their relationship. During the sessions, they worked on issues of privacy, power, intimacy, finances, sex, Mr. Green's retirement and Ms. Green's selfishness. They terminated after eight sessions, feeling better able to deal with Mr. Green's retirement, and their relationship returned to its former equilibrium.

This case highlights the effect of the family network on a woman vulnerable to losses. Ms. Green had first become depressed after her mother's death, again on her daughter's marriage. She then reacted to both her daughter's and her husband's withdrawal as a result of their own situations.

Depression in a Widow

Ms. Gordon, 81, had been sent to a nursing home from the general hospital where her fractured hip had been set. She had fallen over a curbstone while rushing to the funeral of a widower she had been dating. At the nursing home, her behavior was belligerent, she complained of pain and discomfort, and she refused to resume walking. She believed that she was losing control of her mind. She would cry and moan and shake all over, and because she became a management problem, she was sent to a psychiatric hospital for evaluation. On admission, she complained of loneliness. After her husband had died 10 years before, her older sister, also a widow, had moved in with her. Within two months, the two were bickering so much that her sister moved back to a daughter's house. Ms. Gordon kept busy playing cards and Mah-Jongg, attending concerts, and traveling to visit her children and grandchildren. She was meticulous about not being a burden to any of her three children. She had met Mr. Stone only recently; his wife had died six months before. Theirs was a whirlwind courtship, and she was thriving on the excitement of this new relationship. With the unexpected death of Mr. Stone, her world crashed. She felt it was too much to try again to rebuild her life.

Ms. Gordon responded to antidepressant medications. With staff pressure, she resumed walking and joined in group activities; she responded to visits from her children and grandchildren. When she left the hospital, at her children's insistence she hired a housekeeper to stay with her.

Ms. Gordon's case illustrates the destructive impact on the elderly of the death of a lover and friend, the panic resulting in an accident, and the disruption of normal routines as a result of a broken hip.

Alcoholism and Depression in a Single Woman

Ms. Castle, age 70, was admitted with a diagnosis of alcoholism and reactive depression. She had been forced to retire at 65 from her position as an executive assistant. While employed, she had handled her depression by burying herself in her work and enjoying the rewards of her prestigious position. She was involved in numerous organizations and had many friends. She never gave in to the grief she suffered, first at age 16, when her twin sister was killed in an auto accident, then at 24, when her fiancé died of Hodgkin's disease, and in her early 50s on the death of her parents, whom she had supported and to whom she was very attached. After her retirement, she continued to live alone and withdrew from her many activities. She worried that she would not have sufficient income to manage because her retirement pension was marginal and she believed that she was not entitled to social security payments. She began to drink and refused to see anyone. Because she felt she had no right to live and was gradually starving herself to death, a niece arranged for her hospitalization. With Alcoholics Anonymous and other group supports, straightening out social security benefits, and moving to an apartment building for the elderly, Ms. Castle was mobilized to resume her old activity pattern. She joined a group of elderly citizens and took over managing their records, which were in chaos.

Ms. Castle's case illustrates the impact of retirement and financial concerns on a career woman who had managed successfully as long as she was working.

These women of different ages, education, marital status, and socioeconomic backgrounds responded to the proper treatment of their depressions. They were able to readjust their lives and to resume living in a more adaptive fashion. An article by Dr. Samuel Thompson[38] reported on a woman regarded as hopeless at age 60 because of addiction to morphine, barbiturates, sherry, and Scotch. She had been semicomatose, incontinent, belligerent, agitated, abrasive, and confused. Her husband died shortly after her hospitalization. She responded well to long-term psychotherapy, and this woman, now 77, is traveling extensively, does volunteer work with patients in a small emergency-care unit in a general hospital, and is active in other community affairs.

SUICIDE

With the high incidence of depression among the elderly, it is not surprising to find a high incidence of suicide as well. People over 65 are killing themselves at the rate of 5,000–8,000 per year. Although the elderly are 1/10 of the population, they account for 25% of the total number of suicides. The number is probably higher than the reported figure as there are many "hidden" deaths caused by suicidal intent; it is easy for the aged to forget to take life-sustaining medications or mistakenly to take the wrong drug or too many drugs, or to die in a fire caused by smoking in bed. Moreover, the death of an older person is an expected event, and thus, a suicide might go unnoticed. Older people do not usually leave notes. One of two suicide attempts by the elderly is successful, a much higher rate than for other age groups. Adolescents, for example, make seven attempts for every actual suicide.[39]

White males in the 70–74 age group commit suicide at a rate nearly 3 times as high as that of nonwhite men and nearly 5 times as high as that of all women the same age. It appears that the more successful one has been, the harder it is to deal with the irreversible losses of work, spouse, family, and friends. The loss of self-esteem and hope leads to a feeling that life is no longer endurable. The male suicide rate steadily climbs with age; the female rate, although always considerably lower than that for males, peaks at ages 50–54,[39] perhaps a clue to when women experience their greatest losses. Now that women are increasingly engaged in what in the past were considered masculine activities, it is possible that they, too, will be more vulnerable to suicide and in a different pattern than exists at present.

ECONOMIC FACTORS

One of the biggest impacts on the aged is financial stress. More than half of the 23 million people over 65 live on $75 a week. This is particularly true of widowed women, who are the vast majority of aged women in poverty today. Although older people constitute 11% of the total population of the United States, they represent 25% of the poor. The adequacy of income for the elderly varies considerably according to sex, race, and age; whether the individual is living alone or is sharing housing; and whether the individual is employed or has retired. Blacks are twice as likely to be below the poverty line; 36% of the elderly blacks compared with 16% of the elderly white are below the poverty line.[40] The older population is particularly vulnerable to inflation; it is a scourge for those living on fixed incomes; for those who were counting on savings painfully accumulated over many years, but declining steadily in purchasing power; and for those, principally widows, who are losing the struggle to keep up houses that represent a lifetime of savings and who must therefore relocate.

Women experience higher rates of poverty than men at every age, but the differential is greater after 65,[40] particularly for nonmarried elderly women, who are the vast majority. In 1976, the median income for elderly women living alone was $2,900 and for men, $3,400, well below the poverty line. Thus, maintaining independent living arrangements is especially difficult for elderly women, who are more likely than men to live alone.[29]

A move to retirement means a drop of one-half to two-thirds or more in income. Only 2% of retiring women, in contrast to 47% of retiring men, are covered by private pensions, which actually provide only 5% of the total income of people over 65. More women may be covered in the future as women enter the work force earlier and in greater numbers and remain longer now that the compulsory retirement age has been raised to 70. In 1977, women constituted 47% of the work force and were demanding equal rights regarding job assignments, salaries, promotions, pensions, etc.

Current earnings are a relatively small part of the incomes of the elderly, particularly women. In 1970, 40.7% of men 65–69 were in the work force, but only 16.4% of women; of unmarried women 65–69, a higher proportion—20%—supplemented their social security payments with their own earnings. After age 70, these figures drop to 40.7% and 5%, respectively.

At this time, social security is the major source of income for 7 of 10 elderly beneficiaries living alone. Although it pays benefits to 95% of the aged population, it replaces on the average only 58% of the wages of low-income workers and 35% of the wages of high-income workers.[40] Supplementary Security Income (SSI) is available to elderly people who demonstrate need, bringing the combined average income per month to $339. The elderly can also qualify for subsidized housing, whose rents are pegged at 25% of income; for hot lunch programs; for day-care facilities; for special discounts, etc.

In February, 1978, the federal government formally acknowledged the long-criticized inequities for women in the social security system. Women who have been homemakers receive no social security credit at all in their own right. They are entitled to one-half of their retired husband's monthly benefits, but a divorced homemaker cannot live on 50% of her ex-husband's benefit. Divorced homemakers who have been married less than 10 years receive no benefits at all. Widowed homemakers, in order to get benefits, must be at least 50 or be disabled or be caring for children. Women who have worked generally accumulate lower benefits than men because they enter the labor force later, frequently leave earlier (at 62, to care for their retired husbands) and have lower-paying jobs. Benefits for wage-earning couples are calculated on the highest earning, usually the husband's, but this means that a two-earner family may jointly pay more in taxes and collect less in benefits than the single-worker couple.

In addition to a limited income, being "old" means forced unemployment, job discrimination, sex discrimination (in the social security system), poor housing (about 30% of the elderly live in substandard housing), lack of transportation, and, in recent years, crime victimization.

FAMILIES AND THE ELDERLY

Contrary to common perception that adult children frequently abandon their aged parents, data reveal close ties of the elderly to their children and other family members. Shanas found that most children see their elderly parents on a regular basis.[42] Nor are the elderly routinely dumped into institutions. The institutional rate is 5% of the population and has not increased appreciably in recent years.

Families are now the major caretakers of old people who are ill. Shanas reported that in a national survey of older people who were asked to whom, other than their spouses, they would turn in a health crisis, 9 of 10 responded that they would turn to a child. This usually means a daughter, for women traditionally have had the responsibility for aging parents. Sussman[43] reported that married daughters have close ties to their mothers, who in turn are more likely to call on their daughters for help. As the life span increases, so do the numbers of four-generational families, and already there are many reports in the literature of women in their 60s taking care of parents in their 80s and 90s. More and more, women will be responsible for women. Interestingly, although the literature stresses the fact of filial responsibility, there is little evaluation of the quality of the relationships. Whether there is empathy and caring or resentment and annoyance is not elaborated.

LIVING ARRANGEMENTS

In 1975, 38% of women 65 and over were married with the husband present, in contrast to 77% of men who were married and living with their wives; 36% of women over 65 and 41% over 75 lived alone; 22% lived with someone else. Two-thirds of older people, just like younger ones, live in metropolitan areas.

Institutionalization is necessary mainly for the extremely ill and those who do not have families able to take care of them. They include a disproportionate number of the very old, the never-married or widowed, and those who have no children. (One-fourth of women over 70 have no surviving children.) Of the 5% in institutions, 4% are in community nursing homes for the aged and 1% are in mental hospitals.[44] Hospitalization often follows a transient disabling illness when usual coping mechanisms and daily routines are interrupted.

Although the percentage of the elderly in nursing homes is small, the number is still substantial, and the majority are women. In 1977, there were 1,383,600 nursing home beds, 70% of which were filled by women. The preponderance of women is due to their longer life expectancies; to their greater health problems, which limit their ability to be independent; to their greater economic impoverishment; and to their fewer caretakers and social supports. Men turn to their wives in times of sickness, but fewer men nurse their wives when they become ill. These figures represent the number of people in institutions on any given day; it is estimated that one person in four of all those over 65 may enter a long-term facility at some point during their lives.[29] The longer one lives, the greater the chance, as the current median age in institutions is 82. Only 2% of the institutionalized are black because there are fewer older blacks and because of their closer extended-family living arrangments.

There is now an effort to maintain old people in their homes as long as possible, for both humane and economic reasons. The home is seen as the optimal environment for promoting a sense of well-being in the elderly and for reducing memory loss and disorientation. About $13 billion were spent on nursing-home care, with the government paying more than 55% of this amount. With health costs soaring and the number of elderly mounting, the economics of medical care for the older population is a major worry to all. Quality service-supports in the home can be less costly than institutionalization.

ON BEING A SINGLE WOMAN

With the high rate of divorce (one of two marriages), the 70% chance of being a widow after age 65, the increasing numbers of never-married women (from 11 million in 1950 to 20.9 million in 1978) and the ratio of three women to two men after age 65 and of two women to one man by the year 2000, the likelihood of being single or without a husband after age 65 is extremely high. In 1979, there were 13,627,000 women over 65, of whom 828,000 were never married, 7,110,000 were widowed, 448,000 were divorced, outnumbering those married eight to five.

The economic consequences vary with the marital status before age 65. Postmarital women face inequalities in the social security system, whereas, the never-marrieds have longer work histories and probably higher incomes. In 1971, about one fifth of unmarried women, age 65–72, who received social security payments had income from their own earnings.

By not marrying, it is reported that one year is subtracted from the life expectancy rate for each unwedded decade past age 25. Never-married elderly women are also more vulnerable to illness. Studies show that they enter institutions at the rate of 2.6%, compared with a .9% rate for widows. There is also a disproportionately high rate of single women in general hospitals.[46] The lack of family or friends may account for this finding, as hospitalization of the elderly frequently occurs when there is a death or a loss of a supportive relative.[46]

While there is limited research on the sexual behavior of older women, whether single, widowed, or married, there is general agreement that there is no marked difference in sexual aging regardless of marital status, although the never-marrieds show lower levels of sexual activity.[47] In a sample of 71 never-married white women, age 50–69, born from 1890 to 1899, 10 said that they had never wanted to be married, 20 said that they had had some desire for marriage, and 41 reported they would like to have been married. For the most part, these were well-educated women: 16 were high school graduates, and the rest were college graduates or held master's degrees, PhDs, JDs, MDs, etc.[47]

Of these women, one-third reported no overt sexual activity beyond petting and nonorgasm from masturbation, sex dreams, or homosexual experiences. Of the rest, three-quarters had masturbated to orgasm, two-thirds had experienced orgasm, about one-half reported orgasmic dreams, and eight described fairly extensive homosexual contacts. A high degree of success with orgasm was noted, and 21% reported multiple climaxes.[47]

Since the study information was collected in the late 1940s and the early 1950s, when unmarried women were considered spinsters (and often, social misfits), we can assume that today there is a much higher incidence of sexual activity among single women of all ages and that patterns established earlier in life will continue as long as a partner is available.

How Women Cope with Aging

Despite the stresses of bereavement, loneliness, health impairment, and economic privation, many elderly women lead productive and rewarding lives. They are self-sufficient; are living in the community alone or with their spouses, a friend, or a companion; are able to drive; and are maintaining their social networks. Actually, it appears that women are able to handle widowhood more easily than men handle being widowers. Because women have usually been the nurturers and homemakers, they are not totally out of a job at widowhood and can carry on their usual household tasks and responsibilities. For some, widowhood represents a loss of status because their self-esteem was built on the marriage. Whatever the loss of status, however, Cumming stated that the problems of widowhood are more easily resolved than those of retirement. There is not the feeling of failure that frequently accompanies retirement.[48] Surprisingly, many women particularly if provided for financially, come into their own on the death of their husbands. Free of responsibility, they travel and involve themselves in women's clubs, card games, etc.

To a large extent, adaptation is dependent on the cognitive and physical resources that a person can bring to bear on crisis management.[49] Studies of successfully aging individuals indicate that such persons characteristically maintain regular and vigorous physical activities, extensive social contacts, and intellectually and emotionally stimulating pursuits.[50]

The following examples illustrate satisfactory adjustments by women in different age brackets and in different marital states.

A Single Woman of 76

Ms. Pomeroy, a black, single woman in her mid-70s, demonstrates an adaptive response to physical "slowing down" and the onset of failing memory. After graduating from college, Ms. Pomeroy worked for many years at a neighborhood community center planning recreational programs. She was recognized as a leader in the black community, where she struggled to improve the quality of life. At age 65, she was forced to retire. As a volunteer, she organizes numerous discussion and activity groups for black senior citizens and maintains involvement with these programs. With her pension, some savings, and social security payments, she is able to support herself and to maintain her lifestyle with little change, continuing to live alone, to keep up a busy social schedule, and to maintain contact with a wide social network through numerous phone conversations. She keeps up-to-date with newspapers and news broadcasts and is grateful that at age 76 she is able to do so much. Her mind seems clear to her family and friends and her energy level boundless. She herself is very much aware of her tendency to forget as well as her tendency to tire more easily than in years past. She has taken these changes in stride; to compensate, she has learned to write down all engagements and has developed rituals so that she will not forget to take her key, the possibility that worries her the most about her failing memory. When she has an evening event to attend, she rests for an hour before going out. She lives for each day and hopes to maintain this schedule as long as she is physically able.

Ms. Pomeroy demonstrates the importance of developing routines and rituals to compensate for forgetfulness and some physical decline.

A Married Woman of 68

Ms. Peters, a high school graduate, considers herself lucky. She and her husband are in fairly good health and are on good terms with their children and grandchildren. Mr. Peters, age 71, retired from the police force six years ago and works part time for a private security agency. Ms. Peters has continued her part-time job with a catering firm, although now she works only a few times a week helping out at parties. Between Mr. Peters's retirement pension, their social security payments, and their part-time earnings, they are better off financially than in their younger days, when their responsibilities were greater. With their children self-supporting and their mortgage paid, they are free of financial worries. For many years, they had been distressed about their youngest son, who had been on drugs, had been arrested for breaking and entering, and later had been hospitalized after a suicide attempt. At this juncture, he seems to have his life in order, and they no longer feel responsible for getting him straightened out. Ms. Peters has enjoyed helping her children and has welcomed the opportunities to baby-sit and take care of her grandchildren. She is busy cooking and baking their special treats and looks forward to making big family dinners on holidays. Her biggest conflict with her husband has been over his love of fishing. Although he wants her to accompany him, she finds it boring. She figured she had better find some interest of her own, and because she loved to cook, she found her way to the catering firm. Ms. Peters is optimistic about the future. She feels that if their health holds up, she and her husband can have many years of continued happiness.

Ms. Peters is fortunate that she and her husband get along well and enjoy built-in companionship. She has developed her own interests and so has maintained an active life since her children left home and she and her husband have been in semiretirement.

A Widow, Age 84

Widowed at 64, Ms. Locke felt unprepared for all the responsibilities she was forced to take on. She had not finished college and had worked as a secretary for only two years prior to her marriage. With four children to raise, she had devoted herself to her family's needs. She had enjoyed traveling with her husband, taking care of her children, and socializing to a degree. Although she had some interest in playing cards and volunteer activities, her life centered on her husband and family. When the children married and moved out, she and her husband grew even closer to each other, traveling extensively and spending more time together. When her husband died, she was overcome with grief and worry about being on her own. She urged a son who was getting divorced to move in with her, but he refused. Forced to rely on her own resources, she learned to manage a sizable estate, became a volunteer at the local hospital, socialized with her friends, and continued to travel extensively. She wanted to see all the places she hadn't seen "before it was too late." In her 60s she had a sense of wanting to do all the things she either hadn't had time for or hadn't felt free to do. In those days, if she couldn't find a friend to travel with, she felt able to go on her own.

As she reached her 70s many of her friends were dying, and she began to experience periods of depression and stomach difficulties. Although she worried that she too might soon die, she continued to travel until she had cataract surgery at age 76. For a short period then, she began to think about giving up her house and moving into a nursing home. She was conscious of her loneliness and frustrated by her increasing physical weakness. Now that she is in her 80s she is very bothered when at times she draws a blank and is not able to think of a name or an expression or to finish a sentence. At other times, she cannot concentrate on what she is reading. For the past few years, she has had trouble making decisions and feels bad that she needs to lean on others. She is increasingly accepting suggestions and help and is depending more on her children and other relatives for financial advice. She is aware that she worries needlessly and has become pessimistic in her outlook. Any change in her routine requires extra effort, and she is never sure it's worth it. Although she has become indifferent to going out, she usually has a good time when she does. Because most of her friends have died, she socializes very little but continues to visit a friend in a nursing home. She is grateful that she has sufficient funds and an interested family nearby who check on her.

Ms. Locke illustrates the importance of recognizing one's limitations and beginning to accept one's dependency on family and others as a way to adapt.

These women and others have found ways of adapting to and coping with a stage of life that poses many stresses caused by physical decline, the death of family members and friends, changes in lifestyle, changes in social network, and, for some, changes in their financial circumstances. They have developed rituals and routines to compensate for their forgetfulness or their frailties. They have acknowledged some of their dependent needs and seek financial advice or other assistance as necessary.

Many have become involved in local and national organizations, such as the American Association for Retired Persons and the Gray Panthers, an intergenerational, militant movement founded by a woman, Maggie Kuhn, to fight discrimination and prejudice against the elderly. By taking their cause to the media and the Congress, they are reeducating their peers, as well as individuals of all ages, regarding the injustices of the attitudes and policies affecting the elderly. As increasing numbers of women in the population are becoming advocates and lobbyists, their voice is being heard. This productivity and creativity is a striking demonstration of generativity at this stage of the life cycle.

The activist elderly are demanding that social policy be responsive to the needs of this expanding segment of the population. They have already lobbied successfully to raise the compulsory retirement age for most workers to 70. Their next major goal is better health care: more adequate health insurance and revision of the Medicare program to pay for keeping people out of nursing homes and to pay for dentures, eyeglasses, and more drugs. The elderly are campaigning for changes in the social security system: the method of financing, the elimination of limits on outside income, and equity for women.

Crime prevention and compensation for victims affects the elderly, who are victimized by crime, particularly those who live in older, impoverished neighborhoods.

Since most of the elderly are women and many of them live alone, we need to know more about improving their social networks, about helping them to live on reduced incomes, and about preventing their unnecessary institutionalization. We need to know more about the diseases to which women are vulnerable. We need to know more about minority and cross-cultural differences among women and how to reduce the differential in life expectancy and physical health.

The impact that the women's movement will have on the later years of life is still speculative. Now that women are better educated, are having fewer children, are entering the work force in greater numbers (in 1977, 47% of the labor force were women), are divorcing at a rate of one out of two marriages, and are leading alternate lifestyles, such as remaining unmarried but living openly with a man or another woman, it is hard to predict the attitudes and the quality of life after 65 in the years to come.

If women withdraw from their traditional, major caring and nourishing roles in the home, who will take responsibility for the elderly?
If, because of their changing work patterns, women will suffer stress-
related medical problems similar to men's (e.g., heart attacks and high
blood pressure), will their longevity be affected accordingly? The answers to these questions lie in the future.

In conclusion, while some physical decline and minor memory
losses are normal signs of aging, senility and debilitation are not inevitable. One can continue to learn in the 70s and perhaps beyond;
both physical and mental symptoms are usually manageable if properly diagnosed and treated. Women can prepare themselves for their
greater longevity by maintaining physical and social activities, keeping their relationships with family and friends, and continuing their
intellectual pursuits. If a pattern of equanimity, stability, and pur-
posefulness has been established, it will continue through the years.
Although societal attitudes still reflect prejudices against the old, their
increasing numbers and preponderance (by the year 2000, they will
number 31 million) will have a major impact on the social policies of
the future.

REFERENCES

1. Stevenson J: Issues and crises during middlesence, *New York Times*, December 7,
   1977.
2. U.S. Department of Health, Education, and Welfare: Publication No. (HRA) 77-1232;
   Health, United States. Washington, U.S. Government, Printing Office, *1976–77*, p. 4.
3. Neugarten BL: *Middle age and aging*. Chicago, University of Chicago Press, 1968, p.
   14.
4. Cumming E: Further thoughts on the theory of disengagement, UNESCO, *Social
   Science Journal 15*, 377–393, 1963.
5. Siegel JS: Demographic aspects of aging and the older population in the United
   States. U.S. Department of Commerce, Bureau of the Census, Special Studies Series,
   P-23, No. 59, issued May 1976.
6. Parkes MC: Psycho-social transitions: A field for study, *Social Science and Medicine
   Journal 5*:101–115, 1971.
7. Erikson EH: *Childhood and society*. New York, Norton, 1950, p. 232.
8. Cumming E, Henry WE: *Growing old: The process of disengagement*. New York, Basic
   Books, 1961.
9. Butler RN: *Why survive? Being old in America*, New York, Harper & Row, 1975, p. 8.
10. Charatan FB: The psychopathology of old age, *The National Association of Private
    Psychiatric Hospitals Journal 10* (1):31, Fall 1978.
11. Havighurst RJ, Neugarten BL, Tobin SS: Disengagement and patterns of aging, in
    Middle age and aging. Edited by Neugarten BL. Chicago, University of Chicago Press,
    1968, p. 162.
12. National Institute on Aging's Conference on The Older Woman: Continuities and
    Discontinuities, September 14–16, 1978, Bethesda, Md.
13. Weiss RS: National Institute on Aging's Conference on The Older Woman: Continu-
    ities and Discontinuities, September 14–16, 1978, Bethesda, Md.

14. Sontag S: The double standard of aging, *Saturday Review*, September 23, 1972.
15. Goldwyn RM: The woman and esthetic surgery, in *The woman patient*. Vol. 1. Edited by Notman M, Nadelson C. New York, Plenum Press, pp. 271–280, 1978.
16. Kastenbaum R: Getting there ahead of time, *Psychology Today* 5 (7):54, 1971.
17. Perlmutter JF: A gynecological approach to menopause, *The woman patient*. Vol. 1. Edited by Nootman M, Nadelson C. New York, Plenum Press, pp. 323–335, 1978.
18. Renshaw DC: Sex and the senior citizen, *The National Association of Private Psychiatric Hospitals Journal* 10 (1):58, 1978.
19. Masters WH, Johnson VE: *Human sexual response*. Boston, Little, Brown, 1966.
20. Verwoerdt A, Pfeiffer E, Hsioh-Shan W: Sexual behavior in senescence: Changes in sexual activity and interest of aging men and women, *Journal of Geriatric Psychiatry* 2 (2):163–180, 1969.
21. Pfeiffer E, Davis G: Determinants of sexual behavior in middle and old age, *Journal American Geriatric Society* 20:151–158, 1972, p. 56.
22. Christenson CV, Gagnon JH: Sexual behavior in a group of older women, *Journal of Gerontology* 20 (3):351–357, 1965.
23. Busse EW: Aging research: A review and critique, in *Aging: The process and the people*. Edited by Usdin G, Hofling CJ. New York, Brunner/Mazel, 1978.
24. Kaplan H: *The new sex therapy*. New York, Brunner/Mazel, 1974.
25. Berezin MA: Sex and old age: A review of the literature, *Journal of Geriatric Psychiatry*, 2 (2):131–147, 1969.
26. Cleveland WP, Gamturco DJ: Remarriage probability after widowhood: A retrospective method, *Journal of Gerontology* 31:99–103, 1976.
27. Riley MW, Foner A: *Aging and society*, Vol. I, An Inventory of Research Findings, Russell Sage Foundation, New York, 1968.
28. Shanas E, Maddox GL: Aging, health and the organization of health resources, *Handbook Of Aging and the social sciences*, edited by Binstock RH and Shanas E, Van Nostrand Reinhold Co., 1976, p. 594.
29. U.S. Department of Health, Education, and Welfare: Publication No. (HRA) 77-1232; *Health, United States, 1976-77*, p. 15.
30. Summary of Conference on the Older Woman: Continuities and Discontinuities, September 14–16, 1978.
31. U.S. Department of Health, Education, and Welfare: Publication No. (HRA) 77-1232; *Health, United States*, Washington, U.S. Government Printing Office, *1976–77*, p. 10.
32. National Academy of Sciences, Institute of Medicine, Report, 1977.
33. Wells C: *Dementia*. Philadelphia, F. A. Davis, 1971.
34. Butler RN: The future psychiatric care of older people, *The National Association of Private Psychiatric Hospitals Journal* 10 (1):7, 1978.
35. Shanas E, Maddox GL: Aging, health and the organization of health resources, in *Handbook of aging and the social sciences*. Edited by Binstock RH, Shanas E. New York, Van Nostrand Reinhold, 1976, p. 606.
36. Townsend P: The effects of family structure on the likelihood of admission to an institution in old age: The application of a general theory, in *Social structure and the family*. Edited by Shanas E, Streib GF. Englewood Cliffs, N.J., Prentice-Hall, pp. 173–174, 1965.
37. Summary of Conference on The Older Woman: Continuities and Discontinuities, September 14–16, 1978.
38. Thompson PW: The aged, outpatient services, and community mental health programs, *The National Association of Private Psychiatric Hospitals Journal* 10 (1):62–67, 1978.
39. Flaste R: Research begins to focus on suicide among the aged, *The New York Times*, Tuesday, January 2, 1979.

40. Kahne H: *Income maintenance for elderly women: A quality of life prerequisite.* Paper prepared for Conference on The Older Woman: Continuities and Discontinuities, September 14–16, 1978, Bethesda, Md.
41. U.S. Department of Commerce, Bureau of the Census (P60 129), *Money income of families and persons in the United States,* Washington, U.S. Government Printing Office, 1982.
42. Shanas E, Maddox GL: Aging, health, and the organization of health resources, in *Handbook of aging and the social sciences.* Edited by Binstock RH, Shanas E. New York, Van Nostrand Reinhold, 1976, p. 610.
43. Sussman MB: Relationships of adult children with their parents in the U.S., In *Social structure and the family.* Edited by Shanas E, Streib GF. Englewood Cliffs, N.J., Prentice-Hall, 1965.
44. Berkman B: Mental health and the aging: A review of the literature for clinical social workers, *Clinical Social Work Journal 6* (3):231, 1978.
45. U.S. Department of Health, Education, and Welfare: Publication No. (HRA) 77-1232, *Health, United States,* Washington, U.S. Government Printing Office, 1976–77, p. 4.
46. Townsend P: The effects of family structure on the likelihood of admission to an institution in old age: The application of a general theory, in *Social structure and the family.* Edited by Shanas E, Streib GF. Englewood Cliffs, N.J., Prentice-Hall, 1965.
47. Christenson CV, Johnson AB: Sexual patterns in a group of older never-married women, *Journal of Geriatric Psychiatry 6*:80–98.
48. Cumming E: Further thoughts on the theory of disengagement, UNESCO, *Social Science Journal 5*:377–393, 1963.
49. Lipton MA, Nemeroff CB: The Biology of Aging and Its Role in Depression, in *Aging: The process and the people.* Edited by Usdin G, Hofling CJ. New York, Brunner/Mazel, p. 48, 1978.
50. Pfeiffer E: Psychopathology and social pathology, in *Handbook of the psychology of aging,* Edited by Birren JE, Schaie KW. New York, Van Nostrand Reinhold, 1977.

Glossary

These definitions pertain to usage in the text; they are not necessarily complete if used in another context.

Affective: Pertaining to feeling, emotion, or mood.

Affect regulation: The ability to modulate the expression of emotions.

Amenorrhea: The absence of menstrual periods. In *primary* amenorrhea, no menstruation has ever occurred; in *secondary* amenorrhea, menstruation has occurred, then ceased.

Anergic: Lacking energy, passive.

Anorgasmia: A condition in which the individual does not experience orgasm. Origin usually considered psychological.

Anticonvulsants: Drugs that prevent epileptic seizures.

Anxiety: Tension or uneasiness that stems from the anticipation of danger, the source of which is largely unknown or unrecognized. The accompanying physiological changes are similar to those in states of fear. May be regarded as pathologic when so extreme as to interfere with effectiveness in living or reasonable emotional comfort.

Atavistic: Refers to traits, dormant for one or more generations, which reappear in the offspring.

Behavioral psychotherapy: Therapeutic technique based in behavior theory, which postulates that symptoms are learned patterns of behavior that are unadaptive. Therapy is directed to the inhibition and/or extinction of the learned responses.

Borderline personality organization: A psychological diagnostic entity characterized by intense and fluctuating affective states; anger; perception of some people as all good and others as all bad; an inability to form stable, consistent, trusting relationships; and the assignment of one's own feelings to others.

Catharsis: A psychiatric term referring to the therapeutic release of conscious material through talking, or to the release into awareness of repressed material from the unconscious.

Cathexis: The attachment, conscious or unconscious, of emotional feeling and significance to an idea or object, commonly a person.

Character disorder: A personality disorder manifested by a chronic and habitual pattern of reaction that is maladaptive in that it is relatively inflexible, limits the optimal use of potentialities, and often provokes the very counterreactions from the environment that the person seeks to avoid.

Corticoids: Any steroid that has certain chemical or biological properties characteristic of the hormones secreted by the adrenal cortex.

Countertransference: The effects of an analyst's or therapist's unconscious needs and conflicts on his or her understanding or technique. For example, a patient's personality or material may evoke some experience from the therapist's or analyst's past and this may color his or her relationship with the patient.

Defense mechanism: An unconscious psychic mechanism by which an individual handles excessive anxiety caused by conflictual issues.

Delusional: Refers to thinking characterized by delusions, or beliefs not based on realistic perceptions. Delusions arise from unconscious needs and are maintained against logical argument and despite objective contradictory evidence.

Dementia: Loss of intellectual function due to organic impairment.

Denial: A defense mechanism, operating unconsciously, used to resolve emotional conflict and to allay anxiety by disavowing thoughts, feelings, wishes, needs, or external realities that are consciously intolerable.

Depression: This term may refer either to a mood or an affect, or to a specific diagnostic classification. As a mood, it is characterized by feelings of sadness. In the diagnosis of depression are found individual experiences of lowered self-esteem, hopelessness, guilt, and diminished interest in activities. In addition, these mood disturbances may occur with objective signs, for example, apathy, fatigue, loss of appetite, disturbances in sleep, constipation, and difficulty concentrating.

Displacement: A defense mechanism, operating unconsciously, in which an emotion is transferred or "displaced" from its original object to a more acceptable substitute.

Dissociation: A manifestation of confused thought processes and disorganized behavior in which the individual may be at different levels of organization and adaptiveness. We speak of dissociation of ego functions.

Double bind: A name for a type of interaction, noted frequently in schizophrenics' families, in which one member demands a response to a message containing mutually contradictory signals, and the other person is unable to comment on the incongruity or to escape from the situation.

DSM: Abbreviation for the *Diagnostic and Statistical Manual (of Mental Disorders)*, a guide to the nomenclature of psychological disorders.

Dysmenorrhea: The occurrence of pain just before or during menstrual periods.

Dyspareunia: The occurrence of pain during sexual intercourse. The term is usually used in reference to women.

Dysphoric mood: A sense of dissatisfaction or unpleasantness.

Ego: One of the three functional dimensions of the mental apparatus as originally conceptualized by Freud. Ego is the integrative force that mediates between internal impulse or instinct and external reality.

Egocentric: Limited, in outlook or concern, to one's own activities or needs.

Egofunctioning: A psychological theoretical construct; an individual's ability to integrate his or her perceptions and reactions derived from environmental stimuli and internal personal feelings.

Ego regression: A decrease in an individual's previous level of ego functioning.

Ego-syntonic: Describes aspects of an individual's behavior, thoughts, or attitudes he or she views as acceptable and consistent with his or her total personality as opposed to ego-alien. These aspects of behavior may be seen as acceptable or unacceptable by others.

Electroencephalogram (EEG): A graphic recording of the electrical activity of the brain.

Eysenck Personality Inventory: A psychological inventory that has scales for neuroticism and introversion–extroversion.

Grief: The normal, appropriate emotional response to an external and consciously recognized loss; it is usually self-limited and gradually subsides within a reasonable time. To be distinguished from depression.

Hyperemesis gravidarum: Pernicious vomiting in pregnancy.

Hysteria: A term used colloquially in a number of ways, sometimes to connote excessive emotionalism. Technically, it can designate a personality type or an individual who is dramatic, flamboyant, and labile, but not disturbed. Also, a personality disorder characterized by excitability, emotional instability, overreactivity, and dramatization. Individuals with this disorder are often seen as immature, vain, and dependent.

Id: In Freudian theory, that part of the personality structure that harbors the unconscious instinctive desires and strivings of the individual.

Identification: The unconscious process by which an individual patterns himself or herself after another.

Impulse control: The ability to delay and regulate the discharge of sexual and aggressive drives.

Infantilization: The performance of activities or the imposition of rules that are immature or childish.

Introjection: An unconscious mechanism by which a loved or hated external object is symbolically taken into oneself.

Involutional: Refers to the changes or conditions occurring during late middle age in both sexes. The term is becoming outmoded.

Latency age: The period of childhood from ages 6 to 12, when sexual impulses were theoretically considered to be dormant.

Leukorrhea: A whitish discharge from the vagina resulting from inflammation or congestion of the mucous membrane.

Libido: Drive, energy, usually sexual.

Manic: Refers to a condition characterized by excessive elation, irritability, talkativeness, flight of ideas, and accelerated speech and motor activity. When there is a manic-depressive disturbance, manic episodes alternate with depressive episodes.

Masticatory: Refers to the parts of the jaw, including bones, teeth, joints, or ligaments.

Menarche: The onset of menstruation.

Metrorrhagia: Profuse bleeding from the uterus, especially between menstrual periods.

MMPI: The Minnesota Multiphasic Personality Inventory, a standardized, self-rating personality questionnaire consisting of 550 items concerning behavior, feelings, social attitudes, and symptoms of psychopathology.

Monism: The view that reality is one unitary organic whole with no independent parts.

Narcissism: The concentration of psychological interest on the self.

Neonatal: Relating to the newborn during approximately the first month after birth.

Neurasthenia: A term, rarely used in psychiatry today, that was taken literally to mean weakness or exhaustion of the nervous system characterized by chronic fatigue and lack of energy.

Neurosis: An emotional maladaptation characterized by anxiety and arising from unresolved emotional conflicts. This anxiety may be experienced directly or controlled by various psychological mechanisms that may cause other symptoms.

Obsessive-compulsive: A term characterizing the persistent intrusion of unwanted thoughts, urges, or actions that the individual is unable to stop and that may become ritualistic or excessively concerned with conformity and adherence to standards. This term also describes a personality state and the character type of an individual who is rigid, conscientious (sometimes excessively so), and perfectionistic, and who can also be indecisive.

Oedipal (complex, situation, conflict): A set of feelings arising within a family involving attachment of the child to the parent of the opposite sex accompanied by competitive, aggressive feelings toward the parent of the same sex. These feelings are largely repressed because of the fear of displeasure or punishment by the parent of the same sex. In its original use, the term applied only to the male child; it has since been extended to apply to both sexes. The term also represents a maturational development for the child, who is at this time able to relate to both parents in different ways at the same time, rather than to each one primarily as a need-satisfying figure.

Oligomenorrhea: Abnormally scant menstruation.

Oral fixation: An arrest in psychological development at an early period in life, when feeling was primary and attachments to people were dominated by these needs. In adult life, it manifests itself as intense wishes to have all needs gratified.

Paranoid: A disturbance in thinking in which delusions, generally persecutory or grandiose, are the essential abnormality.

Perinatal: Pertaining to the period of childbirth and shortly thereafter; usually beginning with the birth of a fetus of 20 weeks' or more gestation and ending 7–28 days later.

Personality disorder: A group of mental disorders characterized by ingrained maladaptive patterns of behavior, generally lifelong in duration and affecting the entire personality of the individual. When a personality trait becomes disabling or incapacitating, or leads to difficulty in relationships, it is termed a *personality disorder*.

Phobia: An obsessive, persistent, unrealistically intense fear of an object or situation.

Pineal gland: A small, cone-shaped structure in the brain attached to the roof of the third ventricle between the superior colliculi. It produces melatonin, which has an unclear role in reproduction, and is also involved in indolamine metabolism.

Placenta previa: A condition in which the edge of the placenta overlies and partially or completely obstructs the opening of the cervix.

Potentiate: To increase the potential. When used in reference to drugs, the effect that one has on another to increase the potency of each.

Premenstrual tension (distress): Sometimes called *premenstrual syndrome*. The symptoms that sometimes occur just before the menstrual period, including headaches, nausea, psychological tension, and depression.

Projection: A defense mechanism based on the unconscious process of rejecting that which is emotionally unacceptable in the self and attributing those qualities to others.

Pseudocyesis: A condition in which a woman believes that she is pregnant and manifests some of the physical changes that accompany pregnancy when, in fact, she is not pregnant.

Psychoactive drug: When used in reference to psychopharmacological agents, this term refers to any drug (stimulant, depressant, or tranquilizer) with an effect on the mental processes.

Psychoanalytic psychotherapy: Psychotherapy based on psychoanalytic concepts and/or practices, in which association and dreams are traced and the unconscious is explored. The therapy seeks to eliminate or diminish unconscious conflict through conscious awareness and the regarding of old conflicts in terms of adult ego strengths.

Psychodynamics: The systematized knowledge and theory of human behavior and its maturation, the study of which depends largely on the functional significance of emotion. It recognizes the role of unconscious motivation.

Psychogenic: Due to psychological or emotional factors and not to detectable organic or somatic factors.

Psychopathic: Usually used to describe an antisocial personality disorder.

Psychosis: A major mental disorder in which the individual's ability to think, respond emotionally, remember, communicate, interpret reality, and behave appropriately may be so impaired that ordinary life demands cannot be met. It is often characterized by regressive behavior, inappropriate mood, diminished impulse control, and abnormal mental processes, such as delusions and hallucinations.

Psychotropic medication: Any drug with an effect on psychic function, behavior, or experience.

Rationalization: A defense mechanism, operating unconsciously, in which the individual attempts to justify or make consciously tolerable (by plausible means) feelings, behavior, and motives that would otherwise be intolerable.

Reality testing: The ability to appropriately understand, assess, and react to external and internal stimuli.

Regression: The partial or symbolic return to some earlier level of adaptation.

Repression: A defense mechanism, operating unconsciously, in which unacceptable ideas, affects, or impulses are banished from consciousness, or in which those that have never been conscious are kept from becoming conscious.

Schizoid: Refers to a personality disorder manifested by shyness, oversensitivity, seclusiveness, frequent daydreaming, avoidance of close or competitive relationships, and, often, eccentricity. Individuals with this condition often react to disturbing experiences and conflicts with apparent detachment and are often unable to express hostility and aggressive feelings.

Schizophrenia: A form of psychosis manifested by characteristic disturbances of thought, mood, and behavior. Thought disturbances are marked by alterations of concept formation that may lead to misinterpretation of reality and sometimes to delusions and hallucinations. Mood changes include flatness of affect, constriction, inappropriateness, and loss of empathy with others. *Schizophrenia* is sometimes used as a term for a group of related but not identical psychoses.

Separation–individuation: The process of separating from parents and differentiating into an individual, beginning in childhood.

Somatization: The process of converting a mental disorder into physical symptomatology.

Stasis: In psychoanalytic theory, the accumulation of libidinous excitations or tensions because of the blockage of their motor discharge. When the free flow of libido has thus been dammed, stasis results, giving rise to the feeling of anxiety. This is a term used more frequently in older psychoanalytic literature.

Superego: In psychoanalytic theory, that part of the personality associated with ethics, standards, and self-criticism. It is formed by the child's identification with important and esteemed persons in his or her early life, particularly parents. The supposed or actual wishes of these significant persons are taken over as part of the child's own personal standards to help form the "conscience."

Supportive psychotherapy: A technique of psychotherapy that aims to reinforce a patient's defenses and help him or her suppress disturbing psychological material. It utilizes such measures as reassurance, suggestion, inspiration, and education.

Temporal lobe: Part of the cerebral hemisphere which lies laterally and mediates the emotional aspects of behavior and integrates the visual, auditory, and cognitive functions.

Temporomandibular joint: The joint of the jaw.

Tolerance: Increasing resistance to the effects of a drug, so that higher doses are necessary for therapeutic effects.

Transference: In psychoanalytic therapy, the phenomenon of the projection of feelings, thoughts, and wishes from an important figure in the patient's past onto the analyst, who has come to be perceived as that person, transiently or in a more established fashion. The psychiatrist utilizes this phenomenon as a therapeutic tool to help the patient understand his or her emotional problems and their origins.

Vaginismus: Involuntary spasm of the muscles surrounding the vaginal entrance, so that penetration in sexual intercourse is difficult or impossible.

Index